Underground Clinical Vignettes

Surgery

FOURTH EDITION

Underground Clinical Vignettes

Surgery

FOURTH EDITION

Sandra I. Kim, M.D., Ph.D.
Resident in Internal Medicine
Beth Israel Deaconess Medical Center
Harvard Medical School
Boston, Massachusetts

Todd A. Swanson, M.D., Ph.D.
Resident in Radiation Oncology
William Beaumont Hospital
Royal Oak, Michigan

Andrew Z. Wang, M.D.
Resident in Radiation Oncology
Harvard Radiation Oncology Program
Harvard Medical School
Boston, Massachusetts

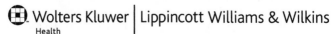
. Wolters Kluwer | Lippincott Williams & Wilkins
Health

Philadelphia · Baltimore · New York · London
Buenos Aires · Hong Kong · Sydney · Tokyo

Acquisitions editor: Nancy Anastasi Duffy
Developmental editor: Nancy Hoffmann
Managing editor: Kelly Horvath
Production editor: Kevin Johnson
Marketing manager: Jennifer Kuklinski
Designer: Doug Smock
Compositor: International Typesetting and Composition

**WO
18.2
K49s
2007**

© 2007 by Lippincott Williams & Wilkins
UCV Step 2 *Surgery*, . . .

Lippincott Williams & Wilkins, a Wolters Kluwer business.

351 West Camden Street   530 Walnut Street
Baltimore, MD 21201   Philadelphia, PA 19106

9 8 7 6 5 4 3 2 1

Library of Congress Cataloging-in-Publication Data

Kim, Sandra.
    Surgery.—4th ed. / Sandra I. Kim, Todd A. Swanson, Andrew Z. Wang.
        p. ; cm.—(Underground clinical vignettes)
    Includes index.
    ISBN-13: 978-0-7817-6847-4
    ISBN-10: 0-7817-6847-0
    1. Surgery—Case studies.   2. Physicians—Licenses—United
States—Examinations—Study guides.   I. Swanson, Todd A.   II. Wang, Andrew Z.
III. Title.   IV. Series.
    [DNLM: 1. Surgical Procedures, Operative—Case Reports.   2. Surgical
Procedures, Operative—Problems and Exercises.   WO 18.2 K49s 2007]
    RD34.B48 2007
    617—dc22

                                                              2007033192

DISCLAIMER
    Care has been taken to confirm the accuracy of the information present and to describe generally accepted practices. However, the authors, editors, and publisher are not responsible for errors or omissions or for any consequences from application of the information in this book and make no warranty, expressed or implied, with respect to the currency, completeness, or accuracy of the contents of the publication. Application of this information in a particular situation remains the professional responsibility of the practitioner; the clinical treatments described and recommended may not be considered absolute and universal recommendations.

    The authors, editors, and publisher have exerted every effort to ensure that drug selection and dosage set forth in this text are in accordance with the current recommendations and practice at the time of publication. However, in view of ongoing research, changes in government regulations, and the constant flow of information relating to drug therapy and drug reactions, the reader is urged to check the package insert for each drug for any change in indications and dosage and for added warnings and precautions. This is particularly important when the recommended agent is a new or infrequently employed drug.

    Some drugs and medical devices presented in this publication have Food and Drug Administration (FDA) clearance for limited use in restricted research settings. It is the responsibility of the health care provider to ascertain the FDA status of each drug or device planned for use in their clinical practice.

To purchase additional copies of this book, call our customer service department at **(800) 638-3030** or fax orders to **(301) 223-2320**. International customers should call **(301) 223-2300**.

Visit Lippincott Williams & Wilkins on the Internet: http://www.lww.com. Lippincott Williams & Wilkins customer service representatives are available from 8:30 am to 6:00 pm, EST.

dedication

Dedicated to the patients we care for.

preface

First published in 1999, the Underground Clinical Vignettes series has provided thousands of students with a highly effective review tool as they prepare for medical exams, particularly the USMLE Step 1 and 2 exams. Designed as a quick study guide, each UCV book contains patient-centered clinical cases that highlight a range of medical diagnoses.

With this new edition of Step 2 Underground Clinical Vignettes, we have incorporated feedback from medical students across the country to provide updated cases with expanded treatment and discussion sections. Every title has more cases, drawing from a broader area within each discipline. A new two-page format enables readers to formulate an initial diagnosis prior to reading the answer to each case. The inclusion of relevant MRI images, x-rays, and photographs allows students to more readily visualize the physical presentation of each case. Breakout boxes, tables, and algorithms have been added, along with twenty all-new, Board-format QAs, making this edition of UCV an ideal source of information for exam review, classroom discussion, and clinical rotations.

The clinical vignettes in this Step 2 series have been revised and updated to reflect current medical thinking on medication, pathogenesis, epidemiology, management, and complications. Although each case presents most of the signs, symptoms, and diagnostic findings for a particular illness, patients typically will not present with such a "complete" picture either clinically or on a medical examination. Cases are not meant to simulate a potential real patient or an exam vignette.

Access to LWW's online companion site, ThePoint, will be offered as a premium with the purchase of the Underground Clinical Vignettes Step 2 bundle. Benefits include an online test link and 160 additional new Board-format questions covering all UCV subject areas.

We hope you will find the Underground Clinical Vignettes series informative and useful. We welcome any feedback, suggestions, or corrections you have about this series. Please contact us at LWW.com/medstudent.

contributors

Series Editors

Sandra I. Kim, M.D., Ph.D.
Resident in Internal Medicine
Beth Israel Deaconess Medical Center
Harvard Medical School
Boston, Massachusetts

Todd A. Swanson, M.D., Ph.D.
Resident in Radiation Oncology
William Beaumont Hospital
Royal Oak, Michigan

Book Editor

Andrew Z. Wang, M.D.
Resident in Radiation Oncology
Harvard Radiation Oncology Program
Harvard Medical School
Boston, Massachusetts

Contributing Editor

Ronald C. Chen, M.D.
Resident in Radiation Oncology
Harvard Radiation Oncology Program
Harvard Medical School
Boston, Massachusetts

Kavid N. Udompanyanan, M.D.
Resident in Emergency Medicine
UCLA/Olive View-UCLA Emergency Medicine Residency
Training Program
Los Angeles, California

Christina L. Boulton, M.D.
Resident in Orthopaedic Surgery
Harvard Combined Orthopaedic Residency Program
Boston, Massachusetts

Surgery Contributors

Abraham Boskovitz, M.D.
Y. Avery Ching, M.D.
Aimee Crago, M.D., Ph.D.
Shivani Gupta, M.D.
Stephanie Misono, M.D., MPH

acknowledgments

Our great thanks to the housestaff and faculty from Beth Israel Deaconess, Massachusetts General Hospital, Brigham and Women's, and Children's Hospital in Boston, whose clinical cases, revisions, and suggestions were indispensable to this series.

Thanks to the editors at Lippincott, especially Nancy Hoffmann who worked overtime on these books.

abbreviations

A-a	alveolar-arterial (oxygen gradient)	ATN	acute tubular necrosis
AAA	abdominal aortic aneurysm	ATPase	adenosine triphosphatase
ABCs	airway, breathing, circulation	ATRA	all-*trans*-retinoic acid
ABGs	arterial blood gases	AV	arteriovenous, atrioventricular
ABPA	allergic bronchopulmonary aspergillosis	AVPD	avoidant personality disorder
		AXR	abdominal x-ray
ABVD	Adriamycin, bleomycin, vinblastine, dacarbazine (chemotherapy)	AZT	azidothymidine (zidovudine)
		BCG	bacille Calmette-Guérin
ACE	angiotensin-converting enzyme	BE	barium enema
ACTH	adrenocorticotropic hormone	BP	blood pressure
ADA	adenosine deaminase, American Diabetic Association	BPD	borderline personality disorder
		BPH	benign prostatic hypertrophy
ADH	antidiuretic hormone	BPK	B-cell progenitor kinase
ADHD	attention-deficit hyperactivity disorder	BPM	beats per minute
		BUN	blood urea nitrogen
AED	automatic external defibrillator	CAA	cerebral amyloid angiopathy
AFP	α-fetoprotein	CABG	coronary artery bypass grafting
AI	aortic insufficiency	CAD	coronary artery disease
AICD	automatic internal cardiac defibrillator	CALLA	common acute lymphoblastic leukemia antigen
AIDS	acquired immunodeficiency syndrome	C-ANCA	cytoplasmic antineutrophil cytoplasmic antibody
ALL	acute lymphocytic leukemia	CAO	chronic airway obstruction
ALS	amyotrophic lateral sclerosis	CAP	community-acquired pneumonia
ALT	alanine aminotransferase	CBC	complete blood count
AML	acute myelogenous leukemia	CBD	common bile duct
AMP	adenosine monophosphate	CBT	cognitive behavioral therapy
ANA	antinuclear antibody	CCU	cardiac care unit
ANCA	antineutrophil cytoplasmic antibody	CD	cluster of differentiation
		CDC	Centers for Disease Control
Angio	angiography	CEA	carcinoembryonic antigen
AP	anteroposterior	CF	cystic fibrosis
aPTT	activated partial thromboplastin time	CFTR	cystic fibrosis transmembrane regulator
ARDS	adult respiratory distress syndrome	CFU	colony-forming unit
ARF	acute renal failure	CHF	congestive heart failure
AS	ankylosing spondylitis	CJD	Creutzfeldt–Jakob disease
ASA	acetylsalicylic acid	CK	creatine kinase
5-ASA	5-aminosalicylic acid	CK-MB	creatine kinase, MB fraction
ASD	atrial septal defect	CLL	chronic lymphocytic leukemia
ASO	antistreptolysin O	CML	chronic myelogenous leukemia
AST	aspartate aminotransferase	CMV	cytomegalovirus
ATLS	Advanced Trauma Life Support (protocol)	CN	cranial nerve
		CNS	central nervous system

CO	cardiac output	ESR	erythrocyte sedimentation rate
COPD	chronic obstructive pulmonary disease	EtOH	ethanol
		FDA	Food and Drug Administration
CPAP	continuous positive airway pressure	Fe_{Na}	fractional excretion of sodium
CPK	creatine phosphokinase	FEV1	forced expiratory volume in 1 second
CPR	cardiopulmonary resuscitation		
CRP	C-reactive protein	FIGO	International Federation of Gynecology and Obstetrics (classification)
CSF	cerebrospinal fluid		
CT	computed tomography		
CVA	cerebrovascular accident	FIo_2	fraction of inspired oxygen
CXR	chest x-ray	FNA	fine-needle aspiration
D&C	dilatation and curettage	FRC	functional residual capacity
DAF	decay-accelerating factor	FSH	follicle-stimulating hormone
DC	direct current	FTA	fluorescent treponemal antibody
DEXA	dual-energy x-ray absorptiometry	FTA-ABS	fluorescent treponemal antibody absorption test
DHEA	dehydroepiandrosterone		
DIC	disseminated intravascular coagulation	5-FU	5-fluorouracil
		FVC	forced vital capacity
DIP	distal interphalangeal (joint)	G6PD	glucose-6-phosphate dehydrogenase
DKA	diabetic ketoacidosis		
DL_{CO}	diffusing capacity of carbon monoxide	GA	gestational age
		GABA	gamma-aminobutyric acid
DM	diabetes mellitus	GABHS	group A β-hemolytic streptococcus
DMD	Duchenne's muscular dystrophy		
DNA	deoxyribonucleic acid	GAD	generalized anxiety disorder
DNase	deoxyribonuclease	GBM	glomerular basement membrane
dsDNA	double-stranded DNA	G-CSF	granulocyte colony-stimulating factor
DTP	diphtheria, tetanus, pertussis (vaccine)		
		GERD	gastroesophageal reflux disease
DTRs	deep tendon reflexes	GFR	glomerular filtration rate
DTs	delirium tremens	GGT	gamma-glutamyltransferase
DUB	dysfunctional uterine bleeding	GI	gastrointestinal
DVT	deep venous thrombosis	GnRH	gonadotropin-releasing hormone
EBV	Epstein–Barr virus	GU	genitourinary
ECG	electrocardiography	HAV	hepatitis A virus
Echo	echocardiography	Hb	hemoglobin
ECMO	extracorporeal membrane oxygenation	HBcAg	hepatitis B core antigen
		HBsAg	hepatitis B surface antigen
EDTA	ethylenediamine tetraacetic acid	HBV	hepatitis B virus
EEG	electroencephalography	hCG	human chorionic gonadotropin
EF	ejection fraction	HCl	hydrogen chloride
EGD	esophagogastroduodenoscopy	HCO_3	bicarbonate
E:I	expiratory-to-inspiratory (ratio)	Hct	hematocrit
ELISA	enzyme-linked immunosorbent assay	HCV	hepatitis C virus
		HDL	high-density lipoprotein
EM	electron microscopy	HEENT	head, eyes, ears, nose, and throat
EMG	electromyography		
ER	emergency room	HELLP	hemolysis, elevated liver enzymes, low platelets (syndrome)
ERCP	endoscopic retrograde cholangiopancreatography		

HEV	hepatitis E virus	LD	Leishman-Donovan (body)
HGPRT	hypoxanthine-guanine phosphoribosyltransferase	LDH	lactate dehydrogenase
		LDL	low-density lipoprotein
HHV	human herpesvirus	LES	lower esophageal sphincter
5-HIAA	5-hydroxyindoleacetic acid	LFTs	liver function tests
HIDA	hepato-iminodiacetic acid (scan)	LH	luteinizing hormone
HIV	human immunodeficiency virus	LHRH	luteinizing hormone–releasing hormone
HLA	human leukocyte antigen		
HPF	high-power field	LKM	liver-kidney microsomal (antibody)
HPI	history of present illness		
HPV	human papillomavirus	LMN	lower motor neuron
HR	heart rate	LP	lumbar puncture
HRCT	high-resolution computed tomography	L/S	lecithin-to-sphingomyelin (ratio)
		LSD	lysergic acid diethylamide
HS	hereditary spherocytosis	LV	left ventricle, left ventricular
HSG	hysterosalpingography	LVH	left ventricular hypertrophy
HSV	herpes simplex virus	Lytes	electrolytes
HUS	hemolytic-uremic syndrome	Mammo	mammography
IABC	intra-aortic balloon counterpulsation	MAO	monoamine oxidase (inhibitor)
		MAP	mean arterial pressure
ICA	internal carotid artery	MCA	middle cerebral artery
ICD	implantable cardiac defibrillator	MCHC	mean corpuscular hemoglobin concentration
ICP	intracranial pressure		
ICU	intensive care unit	MCP	metacarpophalangeal (joint)
ID/CC	identification and chief complaint	MCV	mean corpuscular volume
IDDM	insulin-dependent diabetes mellitus	MDMA	3,4-methylene-dioxymethamphetamine ("Ecstasy")
IE	infectious endocarditis		
IFA	immunofluorescent antibody	MEN	multiple endocrine neoplasia
Ig	immunoglobulin	MGUS	monoclonal gammopathy of undetermined origin
IL	interleukin		
IM	infectious mononucleosis, intramuscular	MHC	major histocompatibility complex
		MI	myocardial infarction
INH	isoniazid	MIBG	metaiodobenzylguanidine
INR	International Normalized Ratio	MMR	measles, mumps, rubella (vaccine)
123-ISS	iodine-123-labeled somatostatin	MPTP	1-methyl-4-phenyl-tetrahydropyridine
IUD	intrauterine device		
IUGR	intrauterine growth retardation		
IV	intravenous	MR	magnetic resonance (imaging)
IVC	inferior vena cava	mRNA	messenger ribonucleic acid
IVIG	intravenous immunoglobulin	MRSA	methicillin-resistant *Staphylococcus aureus*
IVP	intravenous pyelography		
JRA	juvenile rheumatoid arthritis	MS	multiple sclerosis
JVD	jugular venous distention	MTP	metatarsophalangeal (joint)
JVP	jugular venous pressure	MuSK	muscle-specific kinase
KOH	potassium hydroxide	MVA	motor vehicle accident
KS	Kaposi's sarcoma	NADPH	reduced nicotinamide adenine dinucleotide phosphate
KUB	kidney, ureter, bladder		
LA	left atrium	NAME	nevi, atrial myxoma, myxoid neurofibroma, ephilides (syndrome)
LAMB	lentigines, atrial myxoma, blue nevi (syndrome)		

NG	nasogastric	PTT	partial thromboplastin time
NIDDM	non-insulin-dependent diabetes mellitus	RA	rheumatoid arthritis, right atrial
		RBC	red blood cell
NMDA	N-methyl-D-aspartate	RDW	red-cell distribution width
NPO	nil per os (nothing by mouth)	REM	rapid eye movement
NSAID	nonsteroidal anti-inflammatory drug	RF	rheumatoid factor
		RhoGAM	Rh immune globulin
Nuc	nuclear medicine	RNA	ribonucleic acid
OCD	obsessive-compulsive disorder	RPR	rapid plasma reagin
OCP	oral contraceptive pill	RR	respiratory rate
OCPD	obsessive-compulsive personality disorder	RS	Reed-Sternberg (cell)
		RSV	respiratory syncytial virus
17-OHP	17-hydroxyprogesterone	RTA	renal tubular acidosis
OPC	organophosphate and carbamate	RUQ	right upper quadrant
OS	opening snap	RV	residual volume, right ventricle, right ventricular
OTC	over the counter		
PA	posteroanterior	RVH	right ventricular hypertrophy
2-PAM	pralidoxime	SA	sinoatrial
P-ANCA	perinuclear antineutrophil cytoplasmic antibody	SAH	subarachnoid hemorrhage
		SaO_2	oxygen saturation in arterial blood
Pao_2	partial pressure of oxygen		
PAS	periodic acid Schiff	SBE	subacute bacterial endocarditis
PBS	peripheral blood smear	SBFT	small bowel follow-through
Pco_2	partial pressure of carbon dioxide	SC	subcutaneous
		SCC	squamous cell carcinoma
PCOD	polycystic ovary disease	SIADH	syndrome of inappropriate secretion of antidiuretic hormone
PCP	phencyclidine		
PCR	polymerase chain reaction		
PCV	polycythemia vera	SIDS	sudden infant death syndrome
PDA	patent ductus arteriosus	SLE	systemic lupus erythematosus
PE	physical exam	SMA	smooth muscle antibody
PEEP	positive end-expiratory pressure	SSPE	subacute sclerosing panencephalitis
PET	positron emission tomography		
PFTs	pulmonary function tests	SSRI	selective serotonin reuptake inhibitor
PID	pelvic inflammatory disease		
PIP	proximal interphalangeal (joint)	STD	sexually transmitted disease
PKU	phenylketonuria	SZPD	schizoid personality disorder
PMI	point of maximal impulse	T_3	triiodothyronine
PMN	polymorphonuclear (leukocyte)	T_4	thyroxine
PO	per os (by mouth)	TAB	therapeutic abortion
Po_2	partial pressure of oxygen	TB	tuberculosis
PPD	purified protein derivative	TBSA	total body surface area
PROM	premature rupture of membranes	TCA	tricyclic antidepressant
		TCD	transcranial Doppler
PRPP	phosphoribosyl pyrophosphate	TD	tardive dyskinesia
PSA	prostate-specific antigen	TENS	transcutaneous electrical nerve stimulation
PT	prothrombin time		
PTE	pulmonary thromboembolism	TFTs	thyroid function tests
PTH	parathyroid hormone	THC	$trans$-tetrahydrocannabinol
PTSD	post-traumatic stress disorder	TIA	transient ischemic attack

TIBC	total iron-binding capacity	UGI	upper GI (series)
TIPS	transjugular intrahepatic portosystemic shunt	UMN	upper motor neuron
		URI	upper respiratory infection
TLC	total lung capacity	US	ultrasound
TMJ	temporomandibular joint (syndrome)	UTI	urinary tract infection
		UV	ultraviolet
TMP-SMX	trimethoprim-sulfamethoxazole	VCUG	voiding cystourethrogram
TNF	tumor necrosis factor	VDRL	Venereal Disease Research Laboratory
TNM	tumor, node, metastasis (staging)		
		VF	ventricular fibrillation
ToRCH	*Toxoplasma,* rubella, CMV, herpes zoster	VIN	vulvar intraepithelial neoplasia
		VLDL	very low density lipoprotein
tPA	tissue plasminogen activator	VMA	vanillylmandelic acid
TPO	thyroid peroxidase	V/Q	ventilation-perfusion (ratio)
TRAP	tartrate-resistant acid phosphatase	VS	vital signs
		VSD	ventricular septal defect
TRH	thyrotropin-releasing hormone	VT	ventricular tachycardia
TSH	thyroid-stimulating hormone	vWF	von Willebrand factor
TSS	toxic shock syndrome	VZIG	varicella-zoster immune globulin
TSST	toxic shock syndrome toxin	VZV	varicella-zoster virus
TTP	thrombotic thrombocytopenic purpura	WAGR	Wilms' tumor, aniridia, ambiguous genitalia, mental retardation (syndrome)
TUBD	transurethral balloon dilatation		
TUIP	transurethral incision of the prostate	WBC	white blood cell
		WG	Wegener's granulomatosis
TURP	transurethral resection of the prostate	WPW	Wolff–Parkinson–White (syndrome)
UA	urinalysis	XR	x-ray

Underground Clinical Vignettes

Surgery

FOURTH EDITION

case 1

ID/CC An 11-year-old **girl** experiences progressively worsening **shortness of breath** while playing sports (EXERTIONAL DYSPNEA).

HPI Over the past 6 months, she has become increasingly **fatigued** and has recently experienced recurring palpitations.

PE VS: **tachycardia** (HR 120); hypotension (BP 90/60). PE: **no cyanosis**; prominent jugular venous V-wave; **left parasternal heave** (RVH); midsystolic ejection murmur in pulmonic area; **widely split, fixed S₂** (from delayed pulmonic valve closure caused by increased volume in right ventricle); mid-diastolic rumble louder on inspiration (due to increased tricuspid flow); systolic flow murmur at lower left sternal border.

Labs ECG: **atrial fibrillation** (due to atrial dilatation); right axis deviation; **RVH;** incomplete right bundle branch block.

Imaging Echo: RA and RV enlargement; anterior systolic (PARADOXICAL) septal movement with transatrial blood flow. Angio: confirmatory; left-to-right atrial flow; O_2 saturation greater in right ventricle than in superior vena cava.

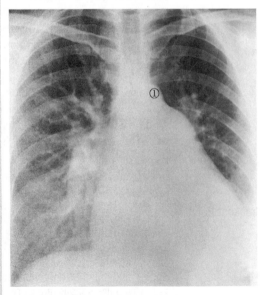

Figure 1-1. CXR: increased pulmonary vascularity (due to left-to-right shunt); dilated pulmonary arteries; right atrium and right ventricle enlarged; small aortic knob (*1*) (due to diminished blood flow).

case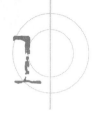

Atrial Septal Defect

Pathogenesis

Atrial septal defects (ASDs) are congenital left-to-right shunts. Three types exist. Approximately 80% of ASDs are **ostium secundum** defects involving the fossa ovalis. They are usually asymptomatic until adulthood, when pulmonary hypertension may develop, converting the left-to-right shunt to a right-to-left shunt (EISENMENGER SYNDROME). **Ostium primum** defects arise inferior to the fossa ovalis and are associated with **AV valve abnormalities** and **Down syndrome.** These commonly present with **heart failure in childhood.** **Sinus venosus** defects arise high in the septum and are associated with anomalous pulmonary venous return.

Epidemiology

More common in females (2:1); **accounts for 30% of congenital heart disease in adults.**

Management

Defect closure via **surgical patching** or transcatheter techniques. Surgery is indicated for ostium secundum defects. Primum defects frequently require repair of mitral valve insufficiency, and sinus venosus defects may need a prosthesis. Contraindications to surgery include small, hemodynamically insignificant defects (ratio of pulmonary flow to systemic flow less than 1:2), long-standing pulmonary hypertension, and Eisenmenger syndrome (may produce postoperative acute heart failure). **The ideal age for surgery is 3 to 6 years.**

Complications

Paradoxic emboli, arrhythmias, heart failure (right-sided), and pulmonary hypertension (especially in primum defects).

Breakout Point

- ASDs are congenital left-to-right shunts that can progress to right-to-left shunts.
- Eisenmenger syndrome is characterized by severe irreversible pulmonary hypertension, and signs of right ventricular failure (elevated jugular venous pressure, hepatic congestion, and pedal edema), cyanosis, and clubbing.

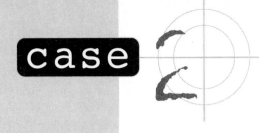

case

ID/CC A 12-year-old **boy** complains of frequent **nose-bleeds.**

HPI Patient often refuses to run with other children, and complains of pain in his legs during activity. He was also found to be hypertensive during the last physical at the school.

PE VS: **BP in arms 180/90** and in **legs 90/60;** no fever; normal RR. PE: no jaundice, pallor, or cyanosis; **harsh, late systolic ejection murmur heard in the interscapular area;** palpable pulsatile collaterals in intercostal spaces; **weak lower-extremity pulses;** neurologic and musculoskeletal exams normal.

Labs CBC: increased hematocrit. ECG: tall R in V_5 and V_6; deep S in V_1 and V_2; LVH.

Imaging CXR: enlarged aortic knob; **rib notching** at the inferior margin of ribs 4 to 9 (collateral circulation).

case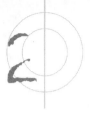

Coarctation of the Aorta

Pathogenesis

Coarctation is usually **distal to the subclavian artery,** resulting in collateral circulation that develops through intercostal arteries leading to pathognomonic rib notching. In the **infantile type,** it is proximal to the ligamentum arteriosum between the subclavian artery and the ductus arteriosus; infants with patent ductus arteriosus (PDA) may have equal upper-extremity and lower-extremity pulses. In the **adult type,** it is distal to the ligamentum arteriosum. The disease may range in severity from heart failure in infants to a lack of symptoms in adolescents and young adults, who are found to have hypertension on routine physicals. Symptomatic patients may complain of **headache,** weakness, **epistaxis,** fatigue, cold legs, intermittent claudication (calf pain while exercising), numbness of the legs, and **differential cyanosis** (unsaturated blood from right ventricle passes to the systemic circulation through the PDA).

Epidemiology

Coarctation of the aorta has a **male** predominance of 2:1 and is associated with **bicuspid aortic valve, Turner syndrome,** VSD, endocardial cushion defect, mitral regurgitation, and PDA.

Management

Control of hypertension; prophylaxis against infectious endocarditis; surgical resection of the stenotic area with an end-to-end anastomosis or grafting, or invasive percutaneous balloon dilatation (BALLOON ANGIOPLASTY).

Complications

Most complications are secondary to hypertension and include cerebral aneurysms, bacterial endocarditis, aortic rupture, heart failure, and aortic dissection.

Breakout Point

- The major clinical manifestation is a **difference in systolic blood pressure** between the upper and lower extremities.
- Classic signs of coarctation of aorta on chest radiographs are **rib notching** and **reverse "3" or "E" sign.**

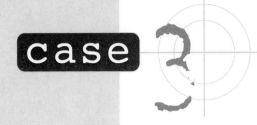

ID/CC   A 3-year-old boy presents with several **syncopal episodes** in which he turned blue.

HPI   **Squatting relieves his symptoms** (increases peripheral vascular resistance, decreasing the right-to-left shunt). His parents also remark that he develops **blue nails and lips** while crying and straining.

PE   VS: tachycardia. PE: small for age; **clubbing** of fingers and toes; **systolic thrill** at left sternal border (due to VSD); parasternal lift (due to RVH); **systolic ejection murmur** (due to pulmonary stenosis); murmur disappears during cyanotic spells (decreased blood flow through pulmonic valve); single S_2 (inaudible P_2 due to pulmonary stenosis).

Labs   CBC: **elevated hemoglobin** (17.4 g/dL) **and hematocrit** (66%); O_2 saturation 72%. ESR elevated. ECG: right axis deviation; RVH.

Imaging   CXR: small heart; rounded, upward-pointing apical shadow with concavity in the region of the main pulmonary artery (BOOT-SHAPED HEART); **diminished pulmonary vascularity** with unusually clear lung fields.

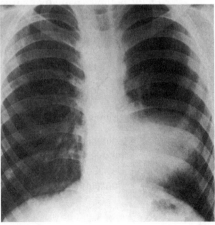

Figure 3-1. Boot-shaped heart with diminished pulmonary vascularity.

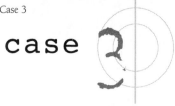

case

Tetralogy of Fallot

Pathogenesis

The etiology of tetralogy of Fallot is unknown; cyanosis results from right-to-left shunting of blood across the VSD. Four defects are involved: large **VSD; RV outflow obstruction** (pulmonary artery stenosis); RVH; and **"overriding" large ascending aorta.** Hypoxic spells with cyanosis may be life-threatening (brain damage). Tetralogy of Fallot is recognizable by cyanosis at or shortly after birth, by the characteristic x-ray findings, and by the pathognomonic **squatting episode** and **cyanotic spell.**

Epidemiology

Tetralogy of Fallot is the **most common congenital cyanotic heart disease.** If left untreated, the mortality rate is 30% at 6 months and 90% to 95% at 20 years. After surgery, 85% of patients live 16 to 28 years.

Management

Treat cyanotic spells with knee-chest position, oxygen, morphine, and beta-blockers. Evaluate with cardiac catheterization before surgical repair. Surgical repair consists of prosthetic closure of the VSD with restoration of RV outflow; **palliative surgery** consists of a shunt construction between the pulmonary and systemic (usually subclavian artery or thoracic aorta) arterial circulation. Pulmonary hypertension is the single most important determinant of success in surgery.

Complications

CHF, ventricular arrhythmias, and sudden death.

Breakout Point

Tetralogy of Fallot

- Stenosis of the pulmonary artery
- Intraventricular communication
- Deviation of the origin of the aorta to the right
- Concentric right ventricular hypertrophy

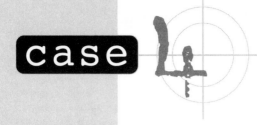
case 4

ID/CC	A surgical consult is called for a **1-day-old** neonate, who seems to **aspirate, cough,** and have **difficulty breathing while feeding.**
HPI	The prenatal screenings and tests were all normal except for **polyhydramnios.** There were no complications during labor.
PE	VS: nl. PE: general—lingering cough. Lung—decreased breath sounds at base of right lung. Heart—RRR, no r/m/g.
Labs	Normal laboratory studies.
Imaging	See Figure 4-1.

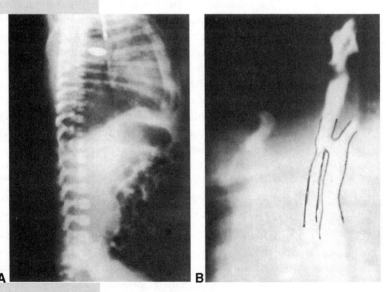

Figure 4-1. A. Lateral radiograph: a small meniscus of barium in the upper pouch. Gas is present in the stomach and intestinal tract. **B.** Another patient: a normal-sized lumen of the esophagus is seen. Dye has spilled into the trachea, outlining the upper trachea and larynx.

case 4

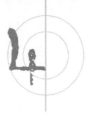

Tracheoesophageal Fistula

Pathogenesis

Tracheoesophageal fistula (TEF) and esophageal atresia (EA) are caused by **improper formation and separation of the trachea and esophagus during development.**

Epidemiology

TEF is a common congenital abnormality and occurs in up to 1 in 3,500 births. When associated with EA, it presents with polyhydramnios during pregnancy.

Management

TEF usually occurs with an EA; thus diagnosis can be achieved by attempting to pass a catheter into the stomach, followed by a **chest radiograph** showing the catheter in an esophageal pouch. TEF without EA can also be visualized on a **swallow study with water-soluble contrast,** but may require a combined **endoscopy** and **bronchoscopy** with direct visualization of methylene blue through the fistulous tract for diagnosis. Once the diagnosis is established, management includes basic supportive measures, such as an infant warmer. Place the infant in a 30- to 40-degree head-up position. Provide intravenous antibiotics for possible aspiration pneumonia. Place a sump suction catheter in the upper pouch to remove the excess secretions and withhold all PO intake. Treatment involves **ligation** of the fistula, in the case of a simple TEF. With EA, primary anastamosis of the esophageal segments is done at the same time, if possible. If the segments are too short, then secondary surgeries may be required with stages including elongation of the esophagus, gastric transposition, or substitution with a segment of colon.

Complications

Inability to feed, aspiration, pneumonia. Surgical complications are rare but may include leakage of the anastamosis, esophageal stricture, recurrent fistula, tracheomalacia, reduced peristalsis, and delayed gastric emptying.

Breakout Point

> Tracheoesophageal fistula is a common congenital abnormality associated with esophageal atresia.

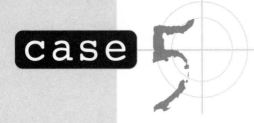

case **5**

PEDIATRIC

ID/CC   A 3-week-old Caucasian boy presents with **projectile vomiting.**

HPI   Patient is the **first-born** child. He was feeding well immediately postpartum, but has developed progressive intolerance of feeds, now vomiting (nonbilious) whatever he eats shortly after meals.

PE   VS: tachycardia. PE: lethargic, dehydrated with dry mucous membranes and no tears. Abdomen is soft with some hyper-resonance and distention over the left upper quadrant with a palpable **"olive-like" mass** in the epigastrium.

Labs   **Hypochloremia, alkalosis (metabolic).**

Imaging   See Figure 5-1.

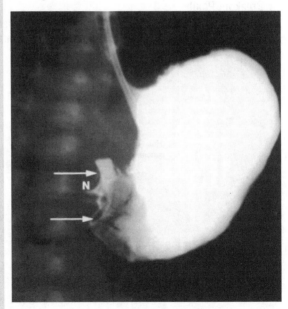

Figure 5-1. Lateral view from barium upper gastrointestinal series showing pyloric channel narrowing (*N*) and elongation with antral shouldering or cushioning.

case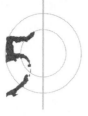

Pyloric Stenosis

Pathogenesis

Pylorc stenosis results from **hypertrophy of the pyloric muscle.** The etiology of hypertrophic pyloric stenosis is unclear. Abnormal nitrous oxide metabolism has been implicated, and a genetic component is suggested by familial cohorts with high rates of pyloric stenosis.

Epidemiology

Incidence of pyloric stenosis is approximately 1 in 3,000 to 4,000. It is more common in patients of Scandinavian descent and in first-born **males** (male-to-female ratio is 4:1 to 5:1).

Management

Initially, correct fluid and electrolyte abnormalities. Surgical repair is curative.

Complications

Severe dehydration, death.

Breakout Point

> Surgical correction is considered the standard of care for all patients with infantile hypertrophic pyloric stenosis.

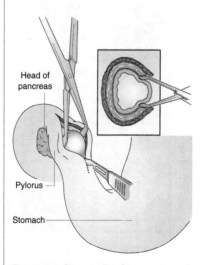

Head of pancreas

Pylorus

Stomach

Figure 5-2. Ramstedt pyloromyotomy for infantile hypertrophic pyloric stenosis.

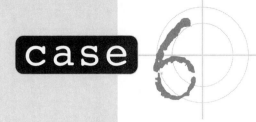

case 6

ID/CC A 40-year-old woman is admitted for **crampy abdominal pain, vomiting, abdominal distention,** and **inability to pass flatus or stool** for the last 12 hours.

HPI She describes a colicky pain that has progressed to severe and sharp pains throughout her abdomen. Of note, she has had **multiple abdominal surgeries,** including an appendectomy, a total abdominal hysterectomy, a cholecystectomy, and most recently, an incisional hernia repair.

PE VS: **tachycardia** (HR 104); tachypnea; no fever. PE: **dry mucous membranes;** abdomen **tympanitic, distended,** and **tender** with no rigidity or rebound tenderness; **bowel sounds high-pitched and increased;** no stool in rectal vault.

Labs CBC: **elevated hematocrit** (due to intraluminal fluid sequestration); elevated WBC count (16,400). Serum and urine amylase slightly increased (modest amylase elevations are seen in intestinal obstruction); lipase normal. ABGs: partially compensated metabolic **acidosis.**

Imaging See Figures 6-1 to 6-3.

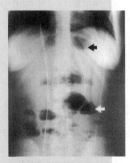

Figure 6-1. Plain upright abdominal film shows multiple **air–fluid levels** in the stomach (*black arrow*), multiple dilated loops of small intestine (*white arrow*), and absence of air in the colon or rectum.

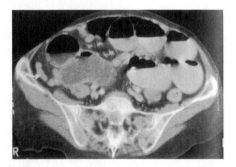

Figure 6-2. CT abdomen: Dilated small bowel loops occupy most of the abdomen. Collapsed distal ileal loops are recognized (*curved arrow*).

11

case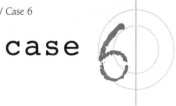

Small Bowel Obstruction (SBO)

Pathogenesis

Mechanical obstruction may be intrinsic (ascaris), extrinsic (hernia ring constricts bowel), or intramural (leiomyoma of wall blocks lumen). The **adynamic** (PARALYTIC) type involves no obstacle but is still considered an obstruction. Pressure increases proximal to the obstruction as fluid and air build up. Over time, the pressure in the lumen may exceed the post-capillary venule pressure, impairing blood flow and eventually producing bowel ischemia and necrosis, leading to perforation. In the United States, the three most common causes of SBO are the **ABCs: adhesions, bulges (hernias), and cancer.** Adhesions (scarring) from prior abdominal surgeries are points of fixation that the small bowel can twist around. Incarcerated or strangulated hernias (e.g., umbilical or inguinal) can also lead to SBO. Cancers can cause an intraluminal obstruction, or result in extraluminal obstruction from inflammation or perforation.

Management

SBO can be **complete or incomplete.** Traditional teaching is to "never let the sun rise or set" on a complete SBO due to the high risk of intestinal necrosis. Patients with a complete SBO are more likely to appear septic, demonstrate no air in the distal colon on radiographic imaging, and have an acute abdomen. These patients should receive immediate resuscitation, nasogastric decompression, and placement of a Foley catheter to measure urine output. An emergent laparotomy is then required to relieve the obstruction. Patients with an incomplete SBO are likely to have a more benign abdominal exam and some air in the colon/rectum on KUB or CT scan. These patients should also receive fluid resuscitation, nasogastric decompression, and a Foley catheter. They can be managed, however, with watchful waiting and serial abdominal exams. If these abdominal exams worsen, or the patients fail to improve, they may then require a laparotomy to relieve the obstruction.

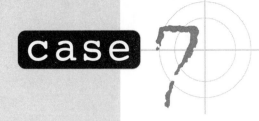

case 7

ID/CC A 55-year-old woman presents with acute onset of severe **abdominal pain, with nausea and vomiting.**

HPI The pain began 6 hours ago, and is diffuse and constant. She also complains of **severe constipation (obstipation)** and abdominal distention. The patient's significant past medical history includes **appendectomy** and **total abdominal hysterectomy** for fibroids.

PE VS: mild tachycardia, afebrile. PE: distended, tympanitic abdomen. Mild tenderness to palpation.

Labs CBC: WBC 12.2K, chemistries normal.

Imaging Abdominal XR: distention of large bowel.

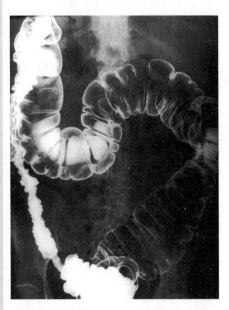

Figure 7-1. Mobile cecum and right colon is readily evident on this air-contrast barium enema.

case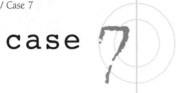

Large-Bowel Obstruction (LBO)

Pathogenesis

This patient has a large bowel obstruction. LBO is an emergency condition that requires early identification and intervention. It is **most commonly seen in the context of advanced colon carcinoma or sigmoid diverticulitis;** less commonly, a sigmoid or cecal volvulus (this case) is present. Obstruction can lead to bowel dilation above the obstruction, leading to bowel edema and ischemia. This can result in perforation, peritonitis, and death.

Epidemiology

Not relevant.

Management

Initial therapy includes volume resuscitation, appropriate preoperative antibiotics, and gastric decompression. Distention of the colon is first treated with **colonoscopic decompression.** In cases where decompression cannot be accomplished or when obstruction recurs, obstruction is treated with cecostomy or more commonly transverse or sigmoid loop **colostomy.** End colostomy with or without a Hartman procedure can be performed.

Complications

Colonic perforation with peritonitis and sepsis.

Breakout Point

> Right-sided colonic lesions can grow quite large before obstruction because of the large caliber of the right colon.

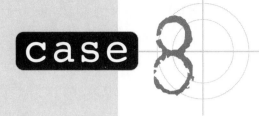

ID/CC   A 32-year-old man complains of **facial flushing** that began following a stressful business meeting; he also complains of recurring severe, throbbing **headaches** (due to increased BP).

HPI   For the past year he has been suffering from **episodic nausea, perspiration, palpitations,** and **anxiety.** He also acknowledges recent obstipation and a **weight loss** of 5 kg over the past 8 months. He is currently asymptomatic. He denies drug use and takes no medications.

PE   VS: no fever (36.4°C); **hypertension** (BP 210/125); normal HR. PE: thin; no arrhythmias; abdominal exam normal.

Labs   Plasma **catecholamines** (epinephrine/norepinephrine) elevated (>2,000 ng/L) at rest; **clonidine** fails to significantly suppress plasma catecholamines; **elevated glucose** (due to increased catecholamines). UA: **elevated** 24-hour **vanillylmandelic acid** (VMA). (Note: Coffee, tea, chocolate, and medications may artificially elevate VMA.)

Imaging   See Figure 8-1.

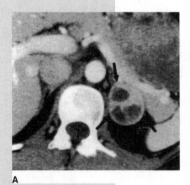

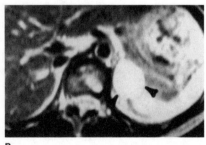

A   **B**

Figure 8-1. A. CT, abdomen. A 3-cm mass is present in the left adrenal gland that contains focal areas of necrosis (*arrows*). **B.** MRT2-weighted MRI scan shows very high signal intensity (*arrowheads*), typical for this diagnosis.

case 8

Pheochromocytoma

Pathogenesis

Pheochromocytomas are **idiopathic primary neoplasms of the chromaffin cells of the adrenal medulla** (derived from **embryonic neural crest cells**) that produce **epinephrine and norepinephrine.** They may also arise from the retroperitoneal, pelvic, or cervical chromaffin bodies of the sympathetic nervous system. The classic triad of symptoms in patients with a pheochromocytoma consists of episodic headache, sweating, and tachycardia. In rare instances, ACTH may be secreted and produce bilateral adrenal hyperplasia and Cushing syndrome.

Epidemiology

Constitutes 0.2% of patients with hypertension and is the **most common adrenal medullary tumor in adults. The rule of 10s** applies: 10% malignant, 10% bilateral, 10% extra-adrenal, 10% calcify, 10% familial, and 10% children. Pheochromocytomas may be a part of **MEN IIa (Sipple) syndrome** (pheochromocytoma, medullary carcinoma of the thyroid, and parathyroid adenoma) and **MEN IIb syndrome** (pheochromocytoma, medullary thyroid carcinoma, and oral and intestinal ganglioneuromatosis) as well as von Hippel–Lindau disease and neurofibromatosis. Isolated pheochromocytomas may also occur in a familial pattern.

Management

Blood pressure control with **phenoxybenzamine or prazosin** (alpha blockade) for 1 to 3 weeks prior to surgery. Chronic volume contraction is controlled with liberal salt intake. **Beta-blockers** are useful in preventing catecholamine-induced arrhythmias and tachycardia, but only after adequate peripheral vasodilation with alpha-blockade. Laparoscopic removal of the tumor is the treatment of choice. **Surgical resection** follows alpha-adrenergic blockade. Close intraoperative and postoperative hemodynamic **monitoring** is indicated to prevent the profound postresection hypotension that results from peripheral vasodilation.

Complications

Cardiac and cerebral damage due to malignant hypertension, cardiomyopathy, CHF, and metastatic disease.

Breakout Point

Clonidine Suppression Test

Clonidine normally suppresses the release of catecholamines from neurons, but does not affect the catecholamine secretion from a pheochromocytoma. Pheochromocytoma is associated with MENIIa and MENIIb.

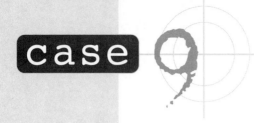

case 9

ID/CC A 24-year-old female reports a **painless mass in the anterior portion of her neck.**

HPI The mass has been present for 2 years but did not grow until recently. As a child, she received **radiotherapy** to the neck. No dysphonia, dysphagia, or dyspnea.

PE VS: normal. PE: **solitary,** nontender, round, **hard mass on right lobe of thyroid** that moves with the gland with swallowing; palpable lymph node on right side of neck (**cervical adenopathy**); remainder of the physical exam is normal.

Labs Calcium, alkaline phosphatase, and serum calcitonin normal; **TFTs normal,** serum thyroglobulin high.

Pathology Fine-needle aspiration of the nodule shows **psammoma bodies.**

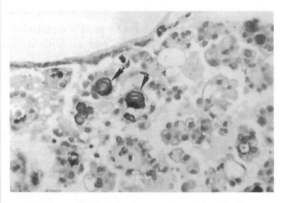

Figure 9-1. Psammoma bodies (*arrows*).

Imaging CXR: normal (no substernal extension or lung masses). US: **solid right lobe thyroid mass** measuring 3 cm. Nuclear scan (technetium-99 pertechnetate isotope): **hypofunctional** (COLD) nodule in right lobe.

case 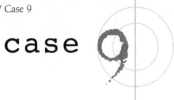 9

Thyroid Cancer

Pathogenesis

This patient has thyroid cancer. Thyroid neoplasms include **carcinomas (papillary, follicular, medullary, or anaplastic)** or **lymphomas.** Patients are usually **euthyroid.** Malignancy is suggested by a **solitary nodule** (versus multinodular goiter), fixation, rapid growth, large size, vocal cord paralysis or hoarseness, hard consistency, and adenopathy. Cold nodules (versus functional or warm ones) are **more likely to be malignant.** Previous **neck irradiation** greatly increases risk of papillary thyroid cancer. The **medullary** type arises in the parafollicular C-cells, is associated with MEN IIa and IIb syndromes, and produces calcitonin.

Epidemiology

4% of U.S. adults have palpable nodules, of which <5% are malignant. The most common thyroid nodules are follicular adenomas, with a 3:1 female-to-male ratio. Among carcinomas, **papillary** is most common, often in young females. It is characterized by early lymphatic metastasis and **slow growth,** with a 95% 5-year survival rate.

Management

Treatment for **papillary, follicular, or medullary** carcinoma is **total or subtotal thyroidectomy.** With lymph node involvement, modified radical neck dissection is indicated. Metastases are treated with postoperative **radioactive iodine** except in the case of medullary carcinoma, in which parafollicular cells do not uptake iodine. **Anaplastic** carcinomas are treated with **radiotherapy** and **chemotherapy,** and possible tracheotomy and thyroidectomy. **Lymphomas** are treated with radiotherapy to neck/superior mediastinum and possible excision if disease is localized.

Complications

Vocal cord paralysis, airway compromise, metastatic disease.

Breakout Point

- Patients with thyroid cancer are often euthyroid even with a palpable thyroid nodule.
- Malignancy is suggested by a solitary nodule (versus multinodular goiter), fixation, rapid growth, large size, vocal cord paralysis or hoarseness, hard consistency, and adenopathy. Cold nodules (versus functional or warm ones) are more likely to be malignant.
- Psammoma bodies are associated with papillary carcinoma.

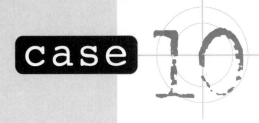

ID/CC A 38-year-old man with a history of **alcoholism** presents to the hospital complaining of **chest pain** after an extensive drinking binge. He reports **multiple bouts of vomiting** before developing a sharp, **tearing chest pain** with **shortness of breath.**

HPI The patient admits having had 12 to 15 drinks prior to episodes of vomiting. He has no other medical problems.

PE VS: temp 38.2°C, HR 137, BP 150/96, RR 28, O₂ sat 95% on room air. HEENT: **subcutaneous crepitus** along anterior neck. Chest: pain (made **worst by neck flexion and swallowing**) over midsternum, lungs clear bilaterally. Heart: tachycardic, regular rhythm, no rubs, murmurs, or gallops. Abdomen: moderate **epigastric pain.**

Labs CBC: initially normal, **WBC elevation** with time; AST: 74, ALT: 36 (ratio > 2:1 indicates alcoholism).

Imaging Conventional radiograph of chest (PA and lateral) and chest CT: **wide mediastinum** with mediastinal and **subcutaneous air** tracking into the neck, **fluid level** in pleural cavity.

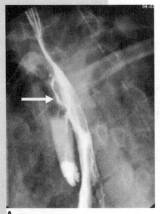
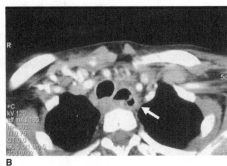

A   B

Figure 10-1. A. Barium small low with water-soluble contrast, such as gastrograffin, and **B.** CT chest can be performed to confirm the diagnosis.

case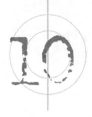

Boerhaave Syndrome

Pathogenesis

This patient has Boerhaave syndrome (ruptured esophagus). Esophageal rupture can result from many causes, the most common being **instrumentation, forceful emesis** (causing increased intraluminal pressures), and **trauma.**

Epidemiology

The mortality of esophageal rupture is approximately 30%, depending on location of perforation, type of injury, health of the patient, and time to diagnosis and intervention. The **left posterior distal esophagus** is the most common location of rupture from forceful emesis, followed by the **right midthoracic** region. Survival is 90% if repaired within 24 hours, but drops to 50% if surgery is delayed.

Management

Antibiotics should be started as soon as possible, with coverage for staphylococcal and streptococcal species, as well as *Pseudomonas* and *Bacteroides.* **Immediate** surgery is needed for essentially all cases. If surgery occurs less than 24 hours after insult, then it is feasible to **primarily close the perforation with external drainage.** If more than 24 hours have passed, primary closure is unlikely to be successful. Alternative treatments must be pursued, such as ligating the esophagus just proximal to the gastroesophageal junction and placing a J-tube for feedings.

Complications

There may be other cofactors leading to esophageal perforation (such as **esophageal cancer, reflux, achalasia, esophageal rings or strictures**), and these should be considered during the workup. **Infection** is the main cause of mortality in these patients.

Breakout Point

Common Features of Boerhaave Syndrome
• Pain
• Vomiting
• Alcoholism
• Gastric ulcers
• Dyspnea
• Shock

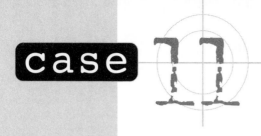

case 11

ID/CC　A **48-year-old** man complains of **difficulty swallowing both solid and liquid foods** (DYSPHAGIA), and a 7-kg **weight loss** over 9 months.

HPI　He states that he frequently **regurgitates** undigested food, especially at night. His dysphagia has **slowly progressed** in severity and frequency over the past year.

PE　VS: normal. PE: **thin; bad breath** (HALITOSIS); abdominal exam unremarkable.

Labs　**Low albumin** (poor nutrition); **ANA** negative; **endoscopy** (to exclude carcinoma) reveals stagnation of food and marked dilatation of esophagus; no strictures; lower esophageal sphincter (LES) hypertonic; biopsy rules out carcinoma; **manometry** reveals **high intraesophageal resting pressure, increased LES pressure,** loss of normal peristaltic waves, and **inadequate LES relaxation after swallowing.**

Imaging　See Figure 11-1.

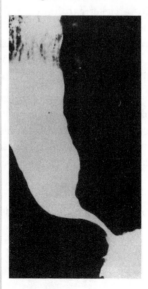

Figure 11-1. "Beak" appearance at the LES on barium swallow.

case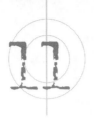

Achalasia

Pathogenesis

Achalasia results from **impaired inhibitory innervation of the Auerbach plexus,** causing defective LES relaxation. Pathogenic theories include a lesion of the dorsal vagus motor nucleus by a neurotropic virus or an esophageal hypersensitivity to gastrin. Achalasia may also present as a paraneoplastic process in older individuals. Also called **cardiospasm,** it characteristically presents with **high LES resting pressure** and **absence of peristaltic contractions** in the body of the esophagus, causing **dysphagia, particularly to cold liquids.**

Epidemiology

Achalasia is uncommon (6 in 100,000), usually occurring in middle age.

Management

Medical management of mild cases with oral nitrates or calcium-channel blockers. Many cases resolve with **balloon dilatation** (cures up to 80% of cases, but beware of perforation). Endoscopic **botulinum toxin injection** into the LES may relieve the obstruction for up to a year. In long-standing disease with marked tortuosity, a Heller **cardiomyotomy** (esophageal muscle incision at the cardioesophageal junction) is effective but can result in gastroesophageal regurgitation; treat with proton-pump inhibitors. Long-term follow-up is always necessary (cancer may develop years later).

Complications

Complications include esophageal carcinoma (**Barrett esophagus**), aspiration pneumonia, abscess, bronchiectasis, pulmonary fibrosis, esophageal ulcerations, and malnutrition. Postsurgical esophageal **reflux** may result in esophagitis and hemorrhage if untreated.

Breakout Point

Signs of Achalasia

- Dysphagia with both liquids AND solids
- Weight loss
- Halitosis
- Undigested regurgitation

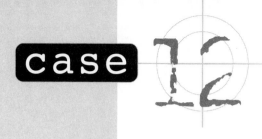

case 12

ID/CC   A 56-year-old man complains of dull, achy **left lower quadrant abdominal pain** with fever, chills, and malaise of 3 days' duration.

HPI   He also complains of recent alternating diarrhea and constipation. The patient admits to a **low-fiber, high-fat diet.**

PE   VS: **tachycardia** (HR 110); normal BP; **fever** (38.3°C). PE: mild dehydration; mild abdominal distention with **left lower quadrant tenderness;** localized voluntary muscle **guarding;** bowel sounds diminished; rectal exam reveals hemorrhoids.

Labs   VS: **tachycardia** (HR 110); normal BP; **fever** (38.3°C). PE: mild dehydration; mild abdominal distention with **left lower quadrant tenderness;** localized voluntary muscle **guarding;** discrete oblong **mass** in left lower quadrant; bowel sounds diminished; rectal exam reveals hemorrhoids; heme-positive stool.

Imaging   KUB: small bowel loop dilatation; increased radio-density in the left lower quadrant.

case 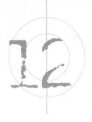 12

Diverticulitis

Pathogenesis

Diverticula are **herniations** of the mucosa and submucosa through the muscular layers of the bowel wall (FALSE DIVERTICULUM) and result from **high intraluminal pressures.** These herniations usually arise at **sites where arterioles traverse the colonic wall** and thus are prone to bleed. These outpouchings may also be obstructed, permitting unabated growth of bacteria and consequent inflammation (DIVERTICULITIS). Diverticulitis has a higher incidence in the left colon (rectosigmoid region) than elsewhere in the GI tract and is **most common in the sigmoid,** where intraluminal pressures are highest. Diverticulitis classically presents as **"left-sided appendicitis."**

Epidemiology

Colonic diverticula occur predominantly in **those older than 50 years.** Risk factors include a **low-fiber diet,** as seen in developed countries. Perforation and consequent generalized peritonitis occur in 10% to 15% of patients.

Management

Treat with **IV fluids, NPO,** and **antibiotics** effective against gram-positive, gram-negative, and anaerobic organisms (e.g., ciprofloxacin plus metronidazole). After an acute episode, a colonic evaluation is needed (one-third of patients have a colonic tumor). Long-term management involves **increased dietary fiber intake** and regular exercise. In cases of recurrent diverticulitis (10% after a single uncomplicated episode and >30% otherwise), patients should consider sigmoidectomy. **Surgery** is indicated in the presence of an abscess (that cannot be drained percutaneously), generalized peritonitis, a fistula, an obstruction, failure of medical therapy, or recurrent episodes.

Complications

Infection may cause necrosis of the colonic wall with **perforation** (microscopically or macroscopically), abscess formation, or peritonitis. Other complications include **obstruction** and **fistula.**

Breakout Point

- Diverticulitis is usually left-sided.
- Uncomplicated diverticulitis is managed with conservative treatment.
- Complicated diverticulitis requires surgical intervention.

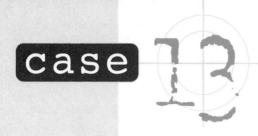

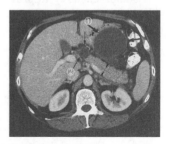

case 13

ID/CC A **42-year-old man** complains of dull, persistent **epigastric** pain.

HPI Pt reports that he has had **fever** for the last 4 days without chills along with **nausea** and scant **vomiting.** Two weeks ago, he was hospitalized for acute gallstone pancreatitis **(previous history).**

PE VS: **fever** (38.5°C); hypertension (BP 140/80); tachycardia (HR 110). PE: alert, active, and in no acute distress; moderate tenderness and a palpable, deep, immotile **mass in epigastric area;** no peritoneal signs.

Labs CBC: moderate **leukocytosis** (15,200/mm³) **with neutrophilia. Mildly elevated blood glucose;** elevated serum **amylase** and **lipase.**

Imaging Abdominal ultrasound shows a **fluid-filled mass** adjacent to the pancreas.

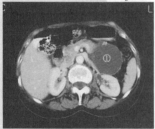

Figure 13-1. CT, abdomen. Fluid-filled cyst (*1*) originating in the pancreatic tail.

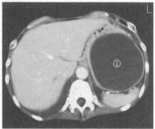

Figure 13-2. CT, abdomen. A different case with large unilecular cyst.

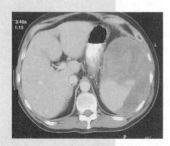

Figure 13-3. CT, abdomen. Hemorrhagic cyst.

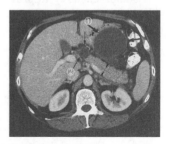

Figure 13-4. CT, abdomen. A different case of large (*1*) and small (*2*) intrapancreatic cysts.

25

case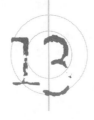

Pancreatic Pseudocyst

Pathogenesis

Most pancreatic pseudocysts occur **following attacks of acute pancreatitis,** when pancreatic secretions fill areas of glandular necrosis, forming compartments of sterile fluid that persist even as inflammation diminishes. Infection of these compartments causes pancreatic abscesses. Pseudocysts **lack an epithelial lining,** while frequently containing high concentrations of pancreatic enzymes. Pseudocysts may also be caused by trauma (most common cause of pseudocysts in children), surgical procedures, and alcohol damage. Pseudocysts are **usually single.**

Epidemiology

Up to 10% of patients with acute pancreatitis develop a pseudocyst.

Management

Cysts >6 cm should be drained after being allowed to **mature 6 weeks. Surgical internal drainage** (anastomosis to internal viscus) is performed most commonly, though **endoscopic** approaches are becoming more common. Signs of pancreatic necrosis or abscess necessitate operative debridement and drainage. **Percutaneous drainage** is preferred for infected cysts. Small cysts (<6 cm) **often regress spontaneously.** Alternative differential diagnoses must be considered as cystic neoplasms can present similarly but should be managed very differently (see Breakout Box).

Complications

Rupture produces peritonitis and is associated with a high mortality. Pseudocysts usually grow rapidly before rupturing. **Infection and bleeding** (intracystic—enlarging mass; intragastric—hematemesis; intraperitoneal—shock) may also occur.

Breakout Point

- Signs of a "pseudo-pseudocyst":
  No hx of pancreatitis
  No previous trauma
  No inflammatory changes on CT
  Internally septated mass/cyst
- Must consider alternate diagnoses!

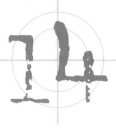
ID/CC A 43-year-old male with a history of alcoholism complains of severe epigastric pain, as well as nausea and vomiting.

HPI The **pain improves** when the patient **assumes the fetal position** or **leans forward**, and worsens with deep breathing and movement. He admits to binge drinking for the last 3 days.

PE VS: **tachycardia** (HR 110); **tachypnea** (RR 28); **fever** (38.6°C); **hypotension** (BP 90/60). PE: agitated and **confused**; dry mucous membranes; decreased breath sounds over left lower lung; **abdomen tender and distended with diminished bowel sounds**; voluntary **guarding** in upper abdomen; mild rigidity without rebound tenderness; ecchymotic discoloration of periumbilical skin (CULLEN SIGN) and over both flanks (GREY–TURNER SIGN); facial muscle spasm when facial nerve is tapped (CHVOSTEK SIGN for hypocalcemia); carpopedal spasm when blood pressure cuff is applied (TROUSSEAU SIGN for hypocalcemia).

Labs **Markedly increased serum and urinary amylase and lipase**. Five of the following **Ranson criteria** present: (1) **on admission:** age >55, leukocytosis >16,000/mm^3, glucose >200, LDH >350, AST >250. (2) **At 48 hours:** >10% hematocrit decrease, >5 mg% increase in BUN, calcium <8, hypoxemia <60, base deficit >4, fluid sequestration <6 L. (3 to 4 signs = 20% mortality; 5 to 6 signs = 40% mortality; >7 signs = 100% mortality).

Imaging CXR: small left **pleural effusion;** basal **atelectasis.** KUB: localized ileus (SENTINEL LOOP); gas in the ascending but not in the transverse colon (COLON CUTOFF SIGN).

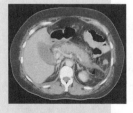

Figure 14-1. CT, abdomen. Edema of the pancreas; peripancreatic stranding (*Standing arrowheads*).

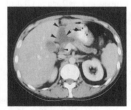

Figure 14-2. A different case with peripancreatic fluid collection.

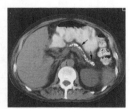

Figure 14-3. CT, abdomen. For comparison, pancreatic atrophy and calcification (*Black arrows*).

27

case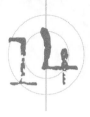

Acute Pancreatitis

Pathogenesis

Pancreatitis is caused mainly by **alcohol abuse** and **gallstones**. Other causes include hyperlipidemia, hypercalcemia, pancreatic tumors, parasitic obstructions (ascaris), collagen vascular diseases, CMV infection (in HIV-positive patients), Legionnaire disease, *Campylobacter*, viral infections, steroids, other medications (e.g., azathioprine, mercaptopurine, and tetracycline), and trauma (ERCP, stomach and gallbladder surgery). Approximately 10% of cases are idiopathic. In gallstone pancreatitis, bile reflux, spasm, or obstruction of the ampulla of Vater may lead to enzyme activation inside the gland with **autodigestion**. Physical signs do not always reflect severity of the disease.

Epidemiology

Annually, between 3 and 6 individuals in 10,000 are affected. Alcohol and biliary disease account for 90% of patients.

Management

Patients should be **NPO** with **nasogastric suction**. Maintain fluid and electrolyte balance; pain control. Give **total parenteral nutrition** if NPO >7 days. Give **antibiotics** if infected bile is suspected. With signs of necrosis, peripancreatic drainage, continuous pancreatic irrigation, subtotal pancreatectomy, or peritoneal lavage may be indicated. IV calcium gluconate should be given if evidence of hypocalcemia and tetany. In gallstone pancreatitis, a cholecystectomy is indicated after the pancreatitis resolves. **Pseudocyst:** if <6 weeks, observe (40% resolve alone); if >6 weeks, open internal drainage. **Abscess:** drain externally via tubes or open-wound technique with lavage under anesthesia every 2 days (BRADLEY).

Complications

DIC, renal failure, ARDS, systemic sepsis, multiorgan systemic failure, toxic psychosis, lactic acidosis, pseudocyst, abscess, septicemia, subcutaneous fat necrosis, and pancreatic exocrine and endocrine insufficiency.

Breakout Point

In addition to the Ranson criteria, the Acute Physiologic and Chronic Health Evaluation (APACHE) scoring system has also been widely used. Several versions of the APACHE scoring system have been utilized, most recently APACHE II through IV.

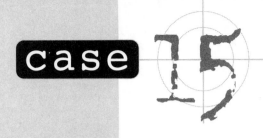

GENERAL SURGERY

ID/CC A 37-year-old **male** CEO presents with **sudden onset** of **severe epigastric pain** and **nausea**.

HPI He **vomited** today and has a 2-week history of intermittent epigastric pain radiating to the back that **worsens with eating**. He works under a great deal of **stress** and drinks 6 cups of **coffee** and several drinks of **alcohol** each day. He also **smokes** 2 packs of cigarettes a day (30-pack-year history) and takes **aspirin** on a regular basis.

PE VS: **fever** (38.7°C); tachycardia (HR 115); **hypotension** (BP 90/50); tachypnea. PE: in **acute distress; diaphoretic**; mild pallor; **abdomen rigid with generalized tenderness** and positive **rebound**; bowel sounds absent; heme-positive stools on rectal exam.

Labs CBC: hemoglobin 12.1 g/dL; **leukocytosis** (18,400/mm^3) **with 85% neutrophils.** Amylase mildly elevated; lipase normal; *Helicobacter pylori* serum antibodies present.

Imaging Chest radiograph: **free subdiaphragmatic intraperitoneal air.**

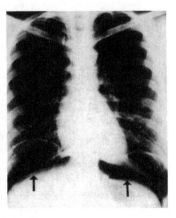

Figure 15-1.

29

case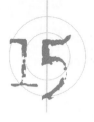

Perforated Peptic Ulcer Disease

Pathogenesis

Gastric ulcers occur when the mucosal barrier is eroded, usually resulting from decreased mucosal resistance. Common causes include **H. pylori** infection, excessive **aspirin and NSAID** use, as well as smoking, alcohol, and steroid use. Duodenal ulcers are associated with acid hypersecretion, whereas gastric ulcers are not. Lesions are **usually single;** 85% of cases are in the **duodenum** (usually within 2 cm of the pylorus); 15% of cases occur in the stomach (usually in the lesser curvature). Lesions may also be found in a gastrojejunal stoma and Meckel diverticulum. Duodenal ulcers generally affect younger patients; gastric ulcers affect older patients, with pain occurring earlier after meals. A complication may be the first manifestation or only vague dyspeptic symptoms may be seen.

Epidemiology

More frequently affects **males,** those with blood group O, patients with chronic liver and lung disease, and individuals with high-carbohydrate, high-protein, low-fiber diets. Perforations develop in 5% of ulcer patients.

Management

Perforation of a gastric ulcer requires a partial gastrectomy and vagotomy, while perforation of a duodenal ulcer requires closure of the perforation, pyloroplasty, and vagotomy. If patient is critical and the ulcer is gastric, treat via closure with an omental patch (GRAHAM PATCH). Laparoscopic perforation closure significantly reduces operative morbidity. **Bleeding** resolves in 75% of cases without operation. Administration of an appropriately broad **antibiotic** regimen (usually ampicillin, metronidazole, and a third-generation cephalosporin) before and after surgery makes a significant difference in clinical improvement. _H. pylori_-associated ulcer disease is treated with a combination of a 10- to 14-day, two- or three-antibiotic regimen combined with a proton-pump inhibitor for 4 to 8 weeks. **Prostaglandin analogs** and **sucralfate** can be used to protect GI mucosa. Active uncomplicated ulcers are treated with proton-pump inhibitors or H_2-receptor blockers alone.

Complications

Complications include **gastric outlet obstruction,** hemorrhage, and malignant change associated with gastric ulcers. Postoperative complications include leakage, hemorrhage, postvagotomy diarrhea, fistula, stomal ulcer, alkaline gastritis, blind loop syndrome, dumping syndrome, and iron and vitamin B_{12} deficiency.

Breakout Point

Common causes of peptic ulcer: H-pylori, aspirin, NSAIDS, smoking, alcohol, steroid use.

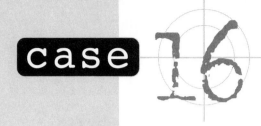
ID/CC A 13-year-old girl on **mechanical ventilation** in the ICU develops acute **respiratory distress**, and bluish coloration of the fingers and tongue (CYANOSIS).

HPI She was **intubated** in the ER 2 days ago following a house fire in which she sustained smoke inhalation injury (with burning of the upper respiratory tract).

PE VS: mild fever (38.3°C); **tachycardia** (HR 125); **hypotension** (BP 80/40); tachypnea. PE: **cyanotic** (late manifestation) and in acute respiratory distress; **tracheal deviation** to the left; poor chest expansion on inspiration, with **hyperresonance** on right (TYMPANITIC); **absence of breath sounds in right lung field; decreased tactile fremitus** in right hemithorax; marked **JVD;** regular rate and rhythm; S_1 and S_2 normal; PMI shifted to left.

Labs CBC: leukocytosis. Lytes/UA: normal. ABGs: **decreased** Po_2 (HYPOXEMIA) and **increased** Pco_2 (HYPERCAPNIA).

Imaging CXR: **hyperlucency** of the right thorax and **mediastinal shift** to the left.

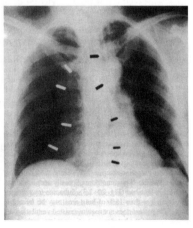

Figure 16-1. Pathology is on the right side (*arrows*) with displacement of mediastinal structures away from it.

case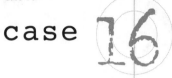

Tension Pneumothorax

Pathogenesis

In a tension pneumothorax, a **one-way valve is established,** permitting air to flow into the pleural space during inspiration without allowing efflux during expiration. Thoracic pressure rises, leading to collapse of the ipsilateral lung, **mediastinal shift and tracheal deviation to the contralateral side,** and severely diminished venous return and contralateral ventilation.

Epidemiology

Trauma and **high-pressure ventilatory support** cause the vast majority of tension pneumothoraces.

Management

Presumptive diagnosis should be based on clinical suspicion; do not wait for x-rays to treat. Life-saving decompression with a **large-bore needle** converts a tension pneumothorax to an open one (associated with less hemodynamic compromise). Insert the needle just above the rib edge (avoiding the neurovascular bundle beneath the rib) in the **second intercostal space** 2 cm lateral to the sternum (in children) or in the midclavicular line (in adults). A **chest tube** should then be placed in the fifth intercostal space, midaxillary line, and directed superiorly.

Complications

Unrecognized tension pneumothorax is associated with respiratory failure, hemodynamic compromise (secondary to decreased venous return), and death. Long-term sequelae are rare after successful treatment.

Breakout Point

- In tension pneumothorax, mediastinal structures including trachea deviate to the contralateral (normal) side.
- Immediate treatment with decompression is life-saving.

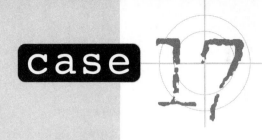
case 17

ID/CC
A 41-year-old man was found on the floor in a **confused and stuporous** state (altered mental status) with "bad breath" (ammonia).

HPI
The patient is a **chronic alcoholic** who binges 3 to 5 times a week. His neighbor reports that he **vomited blood** (HEMATEMESIS; due to esophageal varices) 2 days ago. He has also complained of **severe hemorrhoids.**

PE
VS: no fever; tachycardia (HR 105); hypotension (BP 90/60); no orthopnea; mild tachypnea (RR 20). PE: obtunded, disheveled, and disoriented; dehydrated and **jaundiced; no JVD; parotid enlargement;** fine **flapping tremor of hands** with extension (ASTERIXIS); **spider angiomata; gynecomastia;** muscle wasting; **palmar erythema; caput medusae;** nodular, hard liver palpable 4 cm below costal margin; **bulging, dull flanks** and fluid wave (ASCITES); **splenomegaly; testicular atrophy;** pitting pedal edema.

Labs
CBC: macrocytic, hypochromic **anemia** (Hb 7.1 g/dL); **thrombocytopenia.** LFTs: **AST/ALT ratio 2:1** (alcoholic hepatic damage); **elevated PT, transaminases, GGT, and alkaline phosphatase. Blood glucose low; high blood ammonia;** increased aromatic and decreased branched chain amino acids; **hypoalbuminemia;** liver biopsy shows cirrhosis of the liver (if contraindicated, do peritoneoscopy).

Imaging
Not applicable.

case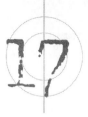

Portal Hypertension

Pathogenesis

This patient has portal hypertension. The etiologies of elevated portal venous pressure (>12 mm Hg, nl 6–8 mm Hg) are classified as **prehepatic** (portal venous occlusion via thrombosis or extrinsic compression), **intrahepatic** (**cirrhosis** [alcoholic, postnecrotic, biliary], hepatitis B and C, hemochromatosis, Wilson disease, and schistosomiasis), and **posthepatic** (constrictive pericarditis and hepatic vein obstruction [Budd–Chiari syndrome]). **Collateral circulation** develops in an effort to decompress the portal system, and **portosystemic anastamoses** are formed as follows: left gastric → azygous (**esophageal varices**); superior → middle and inferior rectal veins (**hemorrhoids**); paraumbilical → inferior gastric (**caput medusae**). Of the many collaterals formed secondary to portal hypertension, severe bleeding is rare except from esophageal varices. Half of all such patients die from this acute event.

Management

Establish **hemodynamic stability.** Treat variceal bleeding with **sclerotherapy** (may cause ulceration and stricture), **octreotide** or **vasopressin,** and **balloon tamponade** (Sengstaken–Blakemore tube). **Surgical shunts** between the portal and systemic circulation decrease portal hypertension but may precipitate encephalopathy. Other treatment modalities include **transjugular intrahepatic portosystemic shunt (TIPS),** splenectomy, devascularization of the lower esophagus (SUGIURA), and **liver transplantation.** Treatment of hepatic encephalopathy includes searching for precipitating factors (dehydration, medications, GI bleed, constipation), reduction of dietary protein, and administration of **neomycin** and/or **lactulose** (to decrease ammonia level).

Complications

Massive **hemorrhage** (secondary to ruptured esophageal varices), **ascites, spontaneous bacterial peritonitis, hepatic encephalopathy, portal vein thrombosis, hypersplenism, and hemorrhoids.**

Breakout Point

Liver Failure Symptoms
• Asterixis
• Jaundice
• Hematemesis
• Altered mental status
• Hemorrhoids
• Cutaneous angiomata

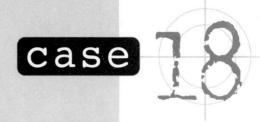
ID/CC A **41-year-old premenopausal (fertile) woman** presents with **right upper quadrant abdominal pain,** associated with **nausea** and **vomiting** that began after she ate an egg-and-avocado salad (fatty foods).

HPI She states that the pain **radiates to the right scapular region** (referred pain). This is the third time such pain has brought this **mother of four** (MULTIPAROUS) to the ER; previous episodes were less intense and spontaneously resolved within a few hours.

PE VS: tachycardia; fever (38.6°C). PE: **obese;** marked tenderness in right upper quadrant with **localized guarding;** gallbladder palpable in subcostal region (30% of cases); **sudden inspiratory arrest** with palpation of right subcostal region (MURPHY SIGN).

Labs CBC: **leukocytosis** (15,500/mm^3). LFTs: bilirubin and alkaline phosphatase slightly elevated; AST and ALT normal; amylase normal.

Imaging On RUQ ultrasound, there is **gallbladder wall thickening (>4 mm), pericholecystic fluid,** and a **sonographic Murphy sign.**

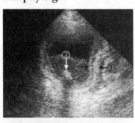

Figure 18-1. US. Thickening of the gallbladder wall (*1*) with gallstones (*2*).

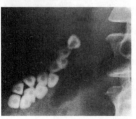

Figure 18-2. XR, abdomen. A different case showing multiple radiopaque gallstones.

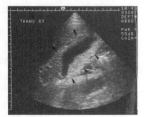

Figure 18-3. US. Another case showing wall thickening with no stones.

GENERAL SURGERY

35

case

Acute Cholecystitis

Pathogenesis

Acute cholecystitis results in the impaction of a gallstone(s) at the cystic–gallbladder junction. If the obstruction is not relieved, subsequent inflammation and edema progress leading to vascular compromise and then ischemia, necrosis, or perforation. There are three types of stones: **cholesterol** (approximately 75%), **black pigment** (associated with hemolysis or cirrhosis), and **brown pigment** (associated with infection). Typically, pain starts after a fatty meal (stimulation of gallbladder contraction leads to impaction of stone in cystic duct or Hartmann pouch, which leads to blockage of bile exit). **Murphy sign,** fever, and leukocytosis suggest a diagnosis of cholecystitis rather than simple biliary colic. **Acalculous** (NO STONES) **cholecystitis** is found in patients with severe debilitating diseases, burns, sepsis, and parasitic (ascariasis) or bacterial (typhoid fever) infections, and less commonly, in those on a prolonged fast or on total parenteral nutrition.

Management

Surgical intervention is often recommended in cases where symptoms began within 72 hours of presentation. Among patients who present later and who respond to medical therapy (NPO, NG tube, IV fluids, and antibiotics), cholecystectomy should be scheduled for 4 to 6 weeks later. If conservative therapy fails, if there is any suspicion of an empyema or perforation, or if acalculous cholecystitis is suspected, emergent cholecystectomy is indicated. **ERCP** may be used to remove common bile duct stones; **cholecystostomy** (percutaneous drainage) may be attempted in high-risk surgical candidates. Gangrenous cholecystitis in elderly patients and diabetics may have a benign presentation.

Complications

Ascending cholangitis should be suspected in the presence of the **Charcot triad** (fever, pain, and jaundice) or **Reynold pentad** (Charcot triad plus shock and mental status alteration). Gallbladder empyema, gallbladder perforation, gallstone pancreatitis, pericholecystic abscess, and cholecystenteric fistulas are other potential complications.

Breakout Point

> The prototypical patient displays the **four Fs: fat, female, forty, and fertile.**

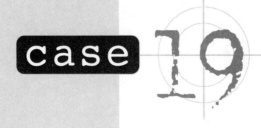

ID/CC A 40-year-old obese male complains of **acute burning and sharp, tearing rectal pain** that began 2 hours ago with **straining** and passage of **hard stool.**

HPI He states that he noticed **blood** on the toilet paper after the bowel movement, and adds that he suffers from chronic **constipation.**

PE VS: normal. PE: unable to find a comfortable position to sit; anorectal exam reveals **sphincter spasm; linear ulceration of the anal mucosa** in posterior midline; **sentinel tag at distal margin of fissure** and **hypertrophic papilla proximal to fissure.**

Labs Not relevant.

Imaging Not relevant.

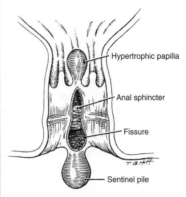

Hypertrophic papilla

Anal sphincter

Fissure

Sentinel pile

Figure 19-1. Associated findings with diagnosis.

case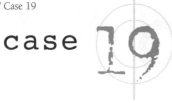

Anal Fissure

Pathogenesis

An anal fissure is a **linear tear in the anorectal mucosa** that is generally caused by **trauma** (from constipation, straining at stool, chronic diarrhea). Other causes include surgical operations in the anorectal area, cathartic abuse, chronic anxiety with spasm of the sphincter, Crohn disease, ulcerative colitis, anal intercourse, syphilis, tuberculosis, and malignancy. Anal fissures may be acute or chronic, and the patient characteristically complains of **minimal bleeding** and **severe pain during stool passage** that may last from minutes to several hours. Chronic fissures present similarly with anal **ulcers, a sentinel pile** (a pouch of skin at the anal verge), and **hypertropic papillae** on exam.

Epidemiology

Anal fissures occur primarily in young and middle-aged adults and show no gender predominance. An increased incidence is seen with receptive anal intercourse and Crohn disease. The condition may also coexist with hemorrhoids and other colorectal diseases.

Management

The vast majority of simple cases respond to medical therapy with **stool softeners, high-fiber diet, analgesics, sitz baths,** and **anesthetic suppositories. Topical nitrates** and **botulinum toxin** have met with some success. In chronic, refractory cases, **lateral internal sphincterotomy** is performed. The fissure itself as well as the pile and papillae may also be resected. If the fissure is not acute, **sigmoidoscopy** should be done to assess the distal colon and rectum, and to evaluate for Crohn disease. Nonhealing ulcers should be biopsied to rule out cancer.

Complications

Chronicity, recurrence, infection, abscess formation, fistulas, contact dermatitis to local anesthetic agents and ointments, postoperative bleeding, urinary retention, chronic mucus discharge, and fecal incontinence (mostly to liquid stool and gas).

Breakout Point

Treatment of Anal Fissures
• Stool softeners
• High-fiber diet
• Anesthetic suppositories
• Topical nitrates
• Botulinum toxin
• Lateral sphincterotomy

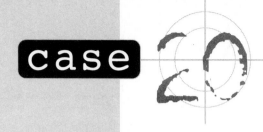

case 20

ID/CC A 49-year-old **man** presents with **intermittent, foul-smelling, purulent anal discharge** that stains his underwear.

HPI The discharge is occasionally accompanied by itching.

PE PE: posterior **opening in the perianal skin** through which a purulent exudate and stool are digitally expressed; irritation of skin surrounding opening; communication between an anal crypt and perianal skin is firm and fibrotic; no fluctuance or tenderness (signs of abscess) noted.

Labs CBC: mild leukocytosis (13,500/mm^3).

Imaging None.

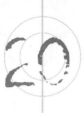

case 20

Anal Fistula

Pathogenesis

An anal fistula is a **fibrous communication between an anal crypt and the perianal skin.** It is usually **secondary to a previous anorectal abscess,** with its origin in anal sinuses. Crohn disease, tuberculosis, trauma, radiation, lymphogranuloma venereum, diverticulitis, and anorectal neoplasia may also cause a fistula. Fistulas may be multiple. The **Goodsall rule** states that fistulas that drain through an opening posterior to a transverse line through the anus (looking at the supine patient from the feet) originate from a posterior midline crypt and take a curved path; anterior fistulas drain anterior crypts and take a straight path. The exception to the Goodsall rule: if the anterior external opening is greater than 3 cm from the anal margin, it usually communicates with the posterior midline crypt.

Epidemiology

Seen predominantly in **males;** most fistulas drain a septic-purulent cavity (ANORECTAL ABSCESS). Fecal incontinence of varying degrees can occur. Also associated with Crohn disease.

Management

Rectosigmoidoscopy must be performed in all cases prior to surgery to assess the terminal colon and rectum. Generally a **barium enema** is also done. **Fistulography** with contrast media may help delineate complex fistulas. Surgery is nearly always indicated due to scarring and chronicity. A **fistulotomy** involves "unroofing" the fistulous tract with marsupialization of borders; **fistulectomy** involves excision of the tract with the surrounding fibrous tissue. A seton (suture run through the fistulous tract that is progressively tightened to induce fibrosis) may be used in some patients. Contraindications to surgery include inflammatory bowel disease and HIV infection.

Complications

Chronicity; spread of infection; malignant degeneration; and puborectalis muscle injury during surgery, leading to incontinence.

Intersphincteric   Transsphincteric   Suprasphincteric   Extrasphincteric

Figure 20-1. Four main types of anal fistulas.

Breakout Point

Additional Studies for Evaluation of Fissures
• Rectosigmoidoscopy
• Barium enema
• Fistulography with contrast
• Transanal ultrasound
• CT scan for anatomy

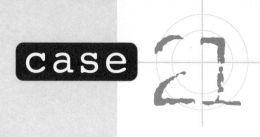

case 21

ID/CC A 19-year-old female presents to the Emergency Room with abdominal pain of 8 hours' duration.

HPI The pain started near the umbilicus but has now **migrated** to the right lower quadrant. She is not hungry (ANOREXIA) and denies any constipation or diarrhea.

PE VS: **tachycardia** (HR 108); normal BP; low-grade fever (38.2°C). PE: abdomen tense with diminished bowel sounds; exquisite tenderness over the **McBurney point** (one-third the distance from the anterior superior iliac spine to the umbilicus); **rebound tenderness** localizing to right lower quadrant; pain on passive extension of hip while lying on left side with knee extended (**PSOAS SIGN**); pain on passive internal rotation of hip (**INTERNAL OBTURATOR SIGN**); right lower quadrant tenderness with deep palpation of left lower quadrant (**ROVSING SIGN**); right side of rectovesical pouch tender on rectal exam. Pelvic exam: normal.

Labs CBC: WBC 14,000/mm^3 with 90% neutrophils. UA: normal. β-HCG: negative.

Imaging See Figures 21-1 and 21-2.

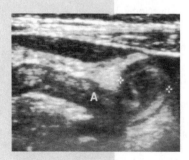

Figure 21-1. Ultrasound. Distended appendix (*A*) with dilated tip *(cursors)*.

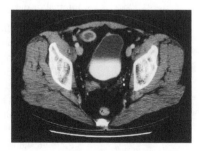

Figure 21-2. Abdominal CT. The thick-walled, fluid-filled appendix with surrounding inflammation.

case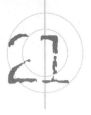

Acute Appendicitis

Pathogenesis

Appendicitis occurs following **obstruction of the appendiceal lumen** as a result of lymphoid hyperplasia, a fecalith, a foreign body, a parasitic infection (ascariasis, amebiasis, trichuriasis), or a stricture. Mucus is secreted into the obstructed lumen, providing a good medium for bacterial growth and inflammation. Additionally, increased luminal and wall pressure leads to ischemia, infarction, and necrosis of the appendix. The appendix may subsequently perforate, causing diffuse peritonitis and sepsis, or it may form an abscess. The appendix may be retrocecal (causing maximal pain in the right lateral, pelvic, or paracolic regions).

Epidemiology

Acute appendicitis is the **most common abdominal surgical emergency;** a diet high in refined sugars and meat is a predisposing factor. The incidence is lower in developing countries and most commonly occurs in patients between the ages of 10 and 30. In elderly patients appendicitis may present only as hypotension.

Management

No analgesics or antibiotics should be administered until a final diagnosis or a decision to operate has been made (withholding analgesics is controversial). **Emergent appendectomy.** Administer postoperative antibiotics that cover gram-positive, gram-negative, and anaerobic organisms (ampicillin + gentamicin + metronidazole). Localized, walled-off abscesses may be treated first with ultrasound-guided or **CT-guided percutaneous drainage** followed by interval or delayed appendectomy 2 to 4 weeks later.

Complications

Complications include pylephlebitis, appendiceal abscess, peritonitis, appendiceal perforation, residual (subphrenic, pelvic) or wall sepsis, and fistula. An incidental carcinoid is found in 1 in 250 appendectomies.

Breakout Point

- All women require a pelvic exam and transvaginal ultrasound to rule out gynecologic etiologies.
- Physical exam findings in acute appendicitis: pain at the McBurney point, rebound tenderness, psoas sign, obturator sign, and Rovsing sign.

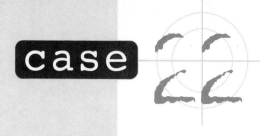

case 22

ID/CC A 60-year-old man presents with several episodes of blood-streaked stools.

HPI The patient also reports **decreased stool caliber,** and a 9-pound weight loss over the last 3 months. He denies any history of hemorrhoids or anal fissures.

PE VS: normal. PE: abdomen soft and nontender; rectal exam reveals a large **mass 5-cm from the anal verge.** The mass is firm and smooth, with a central ulceration. There was bright red blood on examining finger.

Labs CBC: Hgb of 9.5 (mild anemia). LFTs: normal. **Increased CEA** (not specific for colon cancer). **Colonoscopy** showed a mass 8 cm from the **anal verge,** approximately 4 to 5 cm in size, which took up about 40% of the circumference of the lumen; and no other lesions.

Imaging See Figure 22-1. Endorectal coil MRI showed a large apple-core lesion involving the rectum with **transmural invasion** of the right lateral wall of the rectum. A number of presacral lymph nodes within the mesorectal fat appeared abnormal.

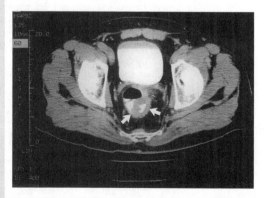

Figure 22-1. CT of the abdomen/pelvis. No lymphadenopathy and no liver metastases were seen. A mass is present in the wall of the rectum (*arrows*).

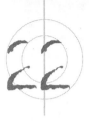

case

Rectal Cancer

Pathogenesis

This patient has rectal cancer. More than 95% of colorectal cancers **progress from a benign neoplastic polyp** to a malignant neoplasm. Although **left-sided** tumors manifest with an early decrease in **stool caliber** and a change in bowel habits along with **obstructive symptoms,** early **right-sided** cancer may be asymptomatic except for **constitutional symptoms** such as fatigue, weight loss, and **anemia,** or melena from occult bleeding. Rectal lesions are also associated with tenesmus and may cause frank rectal bleeding. Risk factors include: familial adenomatous polyposis **(FAP),** hereditary nonpolyposis colorectal cancer **(HNPCC),** history or family history of colorectal cancer, inflammatory bowel disease, diabetes, and alcohol.

Epidemiology

Approximately 150,000 new cases of colorectal cancer are diagnosed each year in the United States, of which two-thirds are colon cancer and one-third are rectal cancer. In the United States, colorectal cancer ranks second to lung cancer as a cause of cancer death, and it is third both in frequency and cause of cancer death among Americans.

Management

Rectal cancers are **staged surgically** (see Appendix A). However, clinical staging is used for management decisions. The workup generally includes colonoscopy (rule out synchronous lesions elsewhere), abdominal/pelvic CT, endorectal ultrasound or endorectal coil MRI (assess the depth of invasion and local lymph node metastases). Surgical resection is the cornerstone of curative treatment. Surgical options are **low anterior resection** (LAR), which preserves the anal sphincter; and **abdominoperineal resection** (APR), which requires a colostomy. Tumors in the upper and middle rectum are managed with LAR. To preserve anal sphincter in distal rectal tumors, neoadjuvant chemoradiotherapy can be given prior to LAR. For very-low-lying rectal cancer, APR followed by possible adjuvant chemoradiation is the treatment of choice.

Complications

Metastatic disease, bowel obstruction, bowel perforation, and abdominal fistulas.

Breakout Point

> Surgical options for rectal cancer are LAR and APR. Patients with stage II or higher rectal cancer need either neoadjuvant or adjuvant therapy.

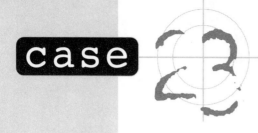

ID/CC A 50-year-old man was found to have a 3-cm **polyp** on his first screening colonoscopy.

HPI The patient has no other significant medical history and has no family history of GI malignancies.

PE Abdominal exam: soft, NT/ND, +BS. No abdominal tenderness or hepatosplenomegaly. Rectal exam was normal, guaiac negative.

Labs CBC: normal. CEA: WNL.

Imaging Abdominal/pelvic CT: no lymphadenopathy or signs of liver metastases.

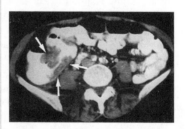

Figure 23-1. CT demonstrates polypoid mass (arrows) filling part of the ascending colon.

case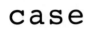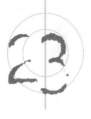

Colon Cancer

Pathogenesis

Most colorectal polyps are adenomatous or hyperplastic, rather than malignant. The risk of colorectal cancer increases with polyp size, number, and histology (e.g., villous worse than tubular architecture).

Epidemiology

Colorectal cancer is the **third most common cancer** in the United States, and is the third leading cause of cancer death in women, the second leading cause of cancer death in men.

Management

The primary and curative treatment for colon cancer is surgical resection. Surgery consists of right or left colectomy and lymph node resection, with primary anastomosis or generation of an ostomy. Adjuvant chemotherapy is based on stage at diagnosis and is given to patients at risk for distant metastatic disease. **Colon cancer screening:** For the average-risk patient, screening starts at **age 50,** and test options include annual fecal occult blood test (FOBT), flexible sigmoidoscopy every 5 years, double-contrast barium enema (DCBE) every 5 years, and colonoscopy every 10 years. For high-risk patients, those with **familial syndromes** (HNPCC, FAP) should be screened with colonoscopy at frequent intervals at an early age. Patients with a first-degree relative with colon cancer or adenomatous polyp diagnosed at age <60 years, or two first-degree relatives diagnosed at any age, should have a screening colonoscopy at age 40 years, or 10 years younger than the earliest diagnosis, and repeated every 5 years. Patients with a first-degree relative with colorectal cancer or adenoma diagnosed at age >60 years; or two or more second-degree relatives with colorectal cancer, should start screening at age 40.

Complications

Metastatic disease, bowel obstruction, bowel perforation, abdominal fistulas, and urinary tract obstruction.

Breakout Point

> Two staging systems are used for colon cancer: the Duke classification, and the TNM staging system of the American Joint Committee on Cancer (AJCC) (see Appendix A).

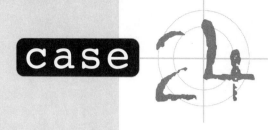

case 24

ID/CC A 69-year-old man presents with **difficulty swallowing** (DYSPHAGIA), started with **solids** and progressed to **liquids**, and **painful swallowing** (ODYNOPHAGIA).

HPI He has a history of gastroesophageal reflux disease (GERD). Before symptoms of dysphagia, he felt food brushing past esophagus. He also reports a 7-kg weight loss over the last 3 months.

PE VS: normal. PE: **nontender left supraclavicular lymph node** (VIRCHOW NODE).

Labs CBC: **decreased hemoglobin** (8.4 g/dL) (anemia from occult bleeding). LFTs: normal AST and ALT. **Heme-positive stool.**

Imaging Both esophagogastroduodenoscopy (EGD) with endoscopic ultrasound (EUS) and colonoscopy were performed. Colonoscopy was normal. EGD showed a fungating and ulcerating mass in the lower third of the esophagus. The mass was partially obstructing, involving about two-thirds of the circumference. It spanned from 35 cm to 39 cm from the incisors. CT of the chest showed thickening of the wall of the distal esophagus, and a lymph node in left supraclavicular area measured 2.7 cm.

Pathology Biopsy results pending.

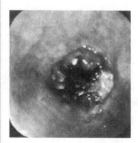

Figure 24-1. Endoscopic view of obstructing esophageal mass.

case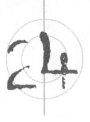

Esophageal Cancer

Pathogenesis

The majority of esophageal cancers are **squamous cell cancers** (SCC) and **adenocarcinomas** (AC). Risk factors associated with SCC are history of **smoking, alcohol** consumption, diet (low in fruits and vegetables, N-nitroso compounds in Asia, betel nut chewing, and very hot foods and beverages), and underlying esophageal disease such as achalasia. ACs are associated with **gastroesophageal reflux** disease, smoking, obesity, and *Helicobacter pylori* infection.

Epidemiology

Esophageal carcinoma occurs in 5 in 100,000 people in the United States. In the past, SCC accounted for 90% of the cases. The incidence for SCC has declined over the last several decades while the incidence for AC has increased to about half of all cases. SCC is usually present in the mid-esophagus, whereas AC generally is present in the lower esophagus.

Management

The staging workup generally includes EGD with EUS, chest CT, and PET-CT. For localized resectable esophageal cancer, patients will undergo neoadjuvant chemoradiotherapy followed by surgical resection. Surgical techniques include **transhiatal esophagectomy, Ivor–Lewis transthoracic esophagectomy, and tri-incisional esophagectomy.** For unresectable disease, definitive chemoradiotherapy is the treatment of choice. Unfortunately, esophageal cancer is a highly lethal disease with a 5-year survival rate around 15%.

Complications

Metastatic disease, occult bleeding, esophageal obstruction, tracheal obstruction, tracheo- and bronchoesophageal fistula, and postoperative leak.

Breakout Point

Risk Factor Differences Between AC and SCC
• Barrett esophagus and chronic reflux are only associated with AC.
• Alcohol is only associated with SCC.
• AC is largely a disease of Caucasians and males.

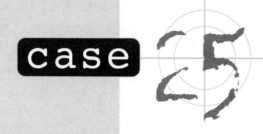

ID/CC A 51-year-old **female** presents with **sudden** onset of **pain** in her right **groin**, nausea and **vomiting**, and a **tense and tender mass** in the groin region.

HPI She was **carrying a heavy box** when the pain began. Over the past several months she has noticed a **bulge** in the right groin that was small and nonpainful. The mass protruded with **exercise/straining**, but it generally disappeared spontaneously.

PE VS: **tachycardia**; normal BP; **fever** (38.1°C). PE: **abdomen slightly distended, tympanitic** (intestine is obstructed with backward accumulation of gas and feces), and tender to palpation; tense, acutely tender, 1.5-cm mass in right groin with changes in skin color below inguinal ligament; mass **does not reduce with pressure**.

Labs CBC: **leukocytosis with neutrophilia.**

Imaging XR, abdomen: a Gastrograffin follow-through study shows **dilated loops of small bowel** secondary to obstruction.

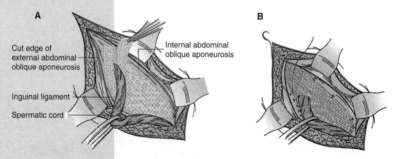

A

Cut edge of external abdominal oblique aponeurosis

Inguinal ligament

Spermatic cord

Internal abdominal oblique aponeurosis

B

Figure 25-1. Lichtenstein hernioplasty, showing placement of the mesh.

case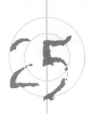

Femoral Hernia

Pathogenesis	Hernia **strangulation** occurs when the constricting hernial ring compromises the blood supply, resulting in **ischemia and necrosis** and possibly leading to **perforation**. The incidence of all hernias and associated strangulation increases with any factor that **increases intra-abdominal pressure**, including obesity, chronic cough, lifting heavy objects, and straining at stool or micturition.
Epidemiology	Femoral hernias **strangulate more** commonly than inguinal or umbilical hernias. Femoral hernias are more common in females than in males, but inguinal hernias are still more common in females (as well as males) than are femoral hernias.
Management	Surgery is the definitive treatment for all hernias. It is **emergently** required if there is strangulated or incarcerated bowel. **Watchful waiting** may be allowed if the patient has minimal symptoms and has close follow-up. The goal of surgery is to repair with minimal tension, which usually involves placing a mesh to patch the defect. The **Shouldice technique** is an open nonmesh repair with incision of all layers of the canal and then reconstruction in four overlapping layers. Open mesh repairs place the mesh in **front** of the defect and laparoscopic repairs place the mesh **behind** the defect. Total extraperitoneal (TEP) repair is the most common laparoscopic procedure, which places the mesh in a **preperitoneal** space, keeping the peritoneum between the mesh and bowel. **Bowel resection** is performed if a segment of nonviable intestine is found.
Complications	May be associated with infection, abscess, hematoma, granuloma formation, and recurrence. Strangulation may lead to **perforation** with generalized **peritonitis**, intra-abdominal abscess formation, or sepsis. Surgery may damage the ileoinguinal nerve, femoral artery, femoral vein, and bladder.
Breakout Point	

Characteristics of Hernias

- Lifetime risk: males 25%, females 5%
- Type: inguinal 95%, femoral 5%
- Inguinal: male-to-female ratio 9:1
- Femoral: female-to-male ratio 4:1

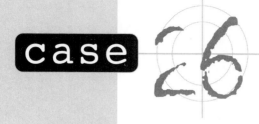
ID/CC A **71-year-old female** nursing-home resident presents with abdominal pain, **nausea, vomiting,** and **inability to pass flatus and stool** (OBSTIPATION) for 3 days.

HPI For the past 3 years she has been having **episodes of "stomach upset"** (biliary colic due to cholelithiasis) that she treats with OTC antacids. She has no history of prior surgery.

PE VS: **tachycardia** (HR 101); low-grade fever (38.1°C). PE: dry oropharynx (due to dehydration from intraluminal third spacing); **abdomen distended, tympanitic, and tender** in all four quadrants; no rebound tenderness; increased bowel sounds; rectal exam unremarkable.

Labs CBC: **moderate leukocytosis with left shift.** LFTs: normal. ABGs: **metabolic alkalosis** (due to vomiting). Lytes: low potassium and chloride.

Imaging See Figure 26-1.

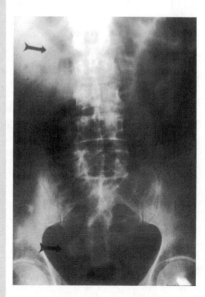

Figure 26-1. Abdominal plain film demonstrating small bowel obstruction. *Arrows* show a gallstone in the right lower quadrant and air in the biliary tree.

case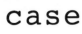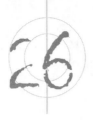

Gallstone Ileus

Pathogenesis

Gallstone ileus results from intestinal obstruction at the level of the ileocecal valve (narrowest portion of small intestine). **Stones formed in the gallbladder gain access to the intestine through a pathologic communication** (FISTULA) between the gallbladder and the intestine (usually the duodenum). These arise as a result of recurrent attacks of gallbladder inflammation with adhesions and scarring. Stones may also pass into the peritoneal cavity, causing extraluminal inflammation and obstruction. Stones that are passed to the GI tract through the biliary ducts are too small to block the ileocecal valve and therefore do not cause gallstone ileus.

Epidemiology

Gallstone ileus is a disease of the **elderly.** There is frequently a delay in diagnosis. Gallstone ileus carries a substantial mortality rate.

Management

Emergent laparotomy with **enterotomy** to extract the stone. Concurrent cholecystectomy and fistula closure may be performed. Palpate to rule out the presence of additional stones prior to closure.

Complications

Recurrence in 10% of cases, perforation, and sepsis.

Breakout Point

Radiographic Findings

- Partial or complete small bowel obstruction
- Air in the biliary tree (pneumobilia)
- Visualization of the stone
- Two adjacent small bowel air–fluid levels in the right upper quadrant

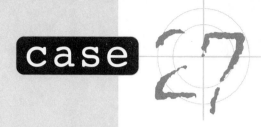
ID/CC A 69-year-old man complains of 6 months of worsening **epigastric pain,** and progressive **loss of appetite.**

HPI He also reports a 5-kg **weight loss** over the last 3 months. The patient has a 40 pack-year **smoking** history, and he drinks 2 beers per night (**alcohol**).

PE VS: normal. PE: pallor; abdominal exam was unremarkable.

Labs CBC: **anemia** (Hb 7.6 g/dL). Stool **heme positive.** LFTs: normal.

Imaging EGD with EUS: a large ulcerating mass in the gastric antrum, biopsy taken. EUS showed tumor invasion into the muscularis propria.

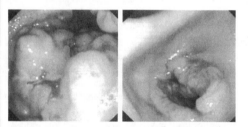

Figure 27-1. EGD: large ulcerating mass in the gastric antrum.

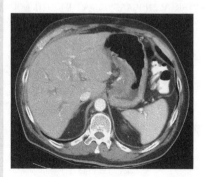

Figure 27-2. CT of the abdomen/pelvis (with oral contrast). A soft-tissue tumor (*T*) in the gastric wall. Note the presence of a lymph node in the gastrohepatic ligament.

GENERAL SURGERY

case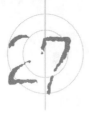

Gastric Cancer

Pathogenesis

Gastric cancer is thought to evolve from chronic inflammation that leads to intestinal metaplasia and dysplasia, and results in adenocarcinoma. Risk factors include **chronic *Helicobacter pylori* infection, pernicious anemia,** a family history of gastric cancer (first-degree relative), diet high in **nitrosamines, smoking,** and **alcohol.** Morphologic types include **ulcerative, polypoid,** superficially spreading (best prognosis), and **diffusely infiltrative (linitis plastica;** worst prognosis). Weight loss and persistent abdominal pain are the most common symptoms. The disease yields deceptively **few symptoms until it is advanced.** Lymphatic spread can lead to a periumbilical nodule (**Sister Mary Joseph node**) or left supraclavicular adenopathy (**Virchow node**). Peritoneal spread can present with an enlarged ovary (**Krukenberg tumor**), or a mass in the cul-de-sac on rectal examination (**Blumer shelf**).

Epidemiology

Gastric cancer is one of the most common cancers worldwide. The highest incidence rates are in Eastern Asia, the Andean regions of South America, and Eastern Europe. North America has one of the lowest rates.

Management

Staging workup for gastric cancer should include EGD with EUS and CT. **Surgical resection** (total or subtotal gastrectomy) with lymph node dissection is the primary curative treatment. Adjuvant chemotherapy and radiotherapy have proven to improve survival. Unfortunately, gastric cancer remains very lethal due to advanced disease at presentation in most patients.

Complications

Fistula to colon, obstruction, bleeding and perforation, and metastatic **disease.**

■ **TABLE 27-1** **GASTRIC ADENOCARCINOMA TUMOR (T), NODE (N), AND METASTASIS (M) STAGING CLASSIFICATION OF THE AMERICAN JOINT COMMITTEE ON CANCER**

Primary Tumor Stage (T)	Definition
Tx	Primary tumor cannot be assessed
T0	No evidence of primary tumor
Tis	Carcinoma in situ: intraepithelial tumor without invasion of the lamina propria
T1	Tumor invades lamina propria or submucosa
T2	Tumor invades muscularis propria or subserosa
T3	Tumor penetrates the serosa without invasion of adjacent structures
T4	Tumor invades adjacent structures
Regional Lymph Nodes (N)	
Nx	Regional lymph nodes cannot be assessed
N0	No regional lymph node metastases
N1	Metastases in 1 to 6 regional lymph nodes
N2	Metastases in 7 to 15 regional lymph nodes
N3	Metastases in more than 15 regional lymph nodes
Distant Metastasis (M)	
Mx	Distant metastases cannot be assessed
M0	No distant metastases
M1	Distant metastases present

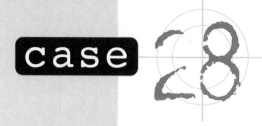

ID/CC A **73-year-old** woman presents with a 3-day history of **dark, tarry stools** (MELENA).

HPI She also reports **fatigue** and mild dizziness. She suffers from hypertension and rheumatoid arthritis, for which she takes **aspirin** daily.

PE VS: **tachycardia** (HR 115); **orthostatic hypotension.** PE: pale; abdomen soft with mild generalized tenderness; no masses; no hepatomegaly or ascites.

Labs CBC: **anemia** (Hb 7.8 g/dL). **BUN increased;** nasogastric tube insertion reveals **"coffee-ground" blood** (blood changes color when exposed to hydrochloric acid); endoscopy shows diffuse erythema and multiple pinpoint **ulcerations** in gastric mucosa in fundus, body, and antrum with no active bleeding.

Imaging Not relevant.

GENERAL SURGERY

case

Upper GI Bleed (UGIB)

Pathogenesis

Upper GI bleeds occur proximal to the ligament of Treitz. **Duodenal ulcers** are the most common cause of UGI bleeds (40%), although **gastric ulcer, erosive gastritis** (hypertrophic, alcoholic, drug-induced), **esophageal varices, Mallory–Weiss tears, and gastric cancer** may be responsible. Other causes include aortoduodenal fistula, AV malformation, stress ulcers (Curling ulcer in burns, trauma), hemobilia, duodenal diverticula, benign tumors, and ruptured aneurysms of the GI tract. Chronic UGI bleeding is associated with iron-deficiency anemia; acute UGI bleeding frequently presents with severe blood volume loss, a normal CBC, hypotension, tachycardia, low urine output, and shock.

Epidemiology

Elderly patients are at especially high risk due to prevalence of NSAID and aspirin use. UGI bleeds are more common in individuals with liver disease, diabetes, and coagulation disorders (such as advanced kidney disease).

Management

Patients should receive **two large-bore IVs** (routine labs, type and cross) and be actively resuscitated with Ringer lactate and packed RBCs. Insert **nasogastric tube** to determine rate and amount of bleeding. Prior to an EGD, patient should receive a **gastric lavage. Endoscopy** is useful both diagnostically and therapeutically (sclerotherapy, coagulation). **Surgery** is indicated if medical treatment fails. In **peptic ulcer disease,** if bleeding is active or if vessels are seen at the ulcer base, **endoscopic control** with epinephrine, polidocanol, cautery, and laser surgery may be attempted; IV proton-pump inhibitors (e.g., omeprazole) reduce the risk of rebleeding. Surgery for bleeding duodenal ulcers usually involves vagotomy and **pyloroplasty;** for severe gastric ulcers, a **gastrectomy** is sometimes performed. **Mallory–Weiss tears** spontaneously achieve hemostasis in 90% of cases. **Hemorrhagic gastritis** is treated with **ice lavage** and **angiographic vasopressin. Varices** require **sclerotherapy** or treatment with **octreotide** or **vasopressin** or transjugular intrahepatic portosystemic shunt **(TIPS).** In cases of hepatic failure, a surgical portosystemic shunt may be indicated.

Complications

Hemorrhagic shock, perforation, peritonitis, aspiration, and cardiac or cerebrovascular ischemia.

Breakout Point

> Most common causes of UGIB: Duodenal and gastric ulcers, gastritis, varices, Mallory-Weiss tears.

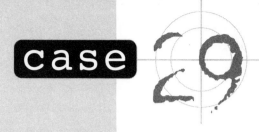

ID/CC A 58-year-old man presents to the ER with **bright red blood per rectum**.

HPI He reports that he has always eaten a **low-fiber diet** and suffers from **chronic constipation**.

PE VS: mild tachycardia; mild hypotension. PE: no acute distress; abdomen soft; **mild tenderness in left lower quadrant** with no masses; no hepatosplenomegaly or ascites; no peritoneal signs; rectal exam reveals frank bright blood in rectal vault; no hemorrhoids.

Labs CBC/Lytes: normal. PT and PTT normal; colonoscopy reveals multiple **diverticula** of left colon; active bleeding from the neck of one.

Imaging See Figures 29-1 and 29-2.

GENERAL SURGERY

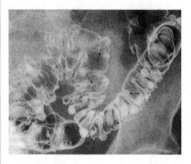

Figure 29-1.
BE (*arrows*).
Diverticular
disease in the
sigmoid colon.
(Common location
due to high intra-
luminal pressure)

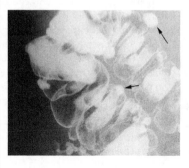

Figure 29-2.
A different case
with diverticular
disease (*arrows*)
of the ascending
colon and appendix.

case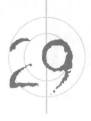

Lower GI Bleed

Pathogenesis

Lower GI bleeding occurs distal to the ligament of Treitz. It is associated with **diverticulosis, AV malformations,** ischemic bowel disease, colon cancer, polyposis, **hemorrhoids,** fissures, inflammatory bowel disease (Crohn disease, ulcerative colitis), Meckel diverticula (ectopic gastric mucosa), coagulopathy, and telangiectasias (Osler–Rendu–Weber). Very brisk bleeds, regardless of site and bleeding, from very distal sites produce hematochezia or bright red blood per rectum; whereas slow, proximal bleeds produce melena.

Epidemiology

Lower GI bleeds occur most commonly in the **elderly.** With severe bleeds, the mortality rate is approximately 10%. Diverticulosis, the most common cause of lower GI bleeding in adults, is associated with a low-fiber diet.

Management

Hemodynamic stabilization and resuscitation should include two large-bore IV catheters, isotonic crystalloid infusions, and packed RBCs or fresh-frozen plasma for coagulation defects. An **anorectal exam** should be performed to rule out hemorrhoids, anal fissures, and other anorectal pathology. Next, an upper GI bleed should be ruled out by passing a **nasogastric tube** to look for blood. If there is evidence of blood, an EGD should be performed. With evidence of bile but no blood in the nasogastric tube, **anoscopy** and/or **sigmoidoscopy** should be performed. With slow bleeds, **colonoscopy** with or without subsequent tagged red cell scans (sensitive for slow bleeds >0.1 mL/min) is usually adequate to establish a diagnosis. Massive bleeds will preclude diagnosis by colonoscopy, so an **angiogram** (sensitive to bleeds >0.5 mL/min) is indicated. **Surgery** is recommended if bleeding is unresponsive to medical treatment or if the patient rebleeds. An exploratory laparotomy with endoscopy and a colectomy may be necessary if the source of bleeding cannot be determined. **Diverticulosis:** asymptomatic diverticulosis is managed with a **high-fiber diet.** Anticholinergics, antidepressants, and antibiotics have no proven effect.

Complications

Shock and death.

Breakout Point

Always rule out upper GI bleed in the setting of suspected lower GI bleed.

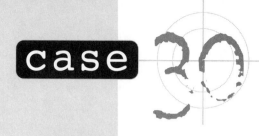

case 30

ID/CC A 27-year-old woman presents with an extremely tender **anal mass** associated with **acute perianal pain** and **bright red blood** on bathroom tissue after wiping.

HPI The patient is a **smoker** and reports a high-fat, **low-fiber diet.** She has a history of **chronic constipation,** anorectal pruritus, and grade II hemorrhoids (protrusion with defecation, spontaneous reduction).

PE VS: normal. PE: rectal exam reveals a small, **well-defined, rounded, painful, purplish-red, firm mass** in anal margin with peripheral swelling (venous clot surrounded by inflammation).

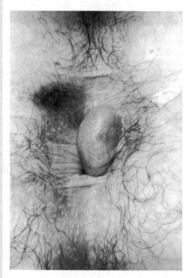

Figure 30-1. Thrombosed external mass.

Labs Proctoscopy: no rectal masses.

Imaging Not relevant.

case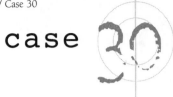

Hemorrhoids

Pathogenesis

Hemorrhoids are submucosal **venous dilatations** that may arise with increased **intra-abdominal pressure,** as occurs with straining on defecation or prolonged sitting or standing (associated with increased hydrostatic pressure). External hemorrhoids **arise distal to the dentate line** and may thrombose, causing acute pain and inflammation. These are often aggravated by consumption of spicy food, alcohol, chronic diarrhea, and anal infections. Internal hemorrhoids are vascular anal connective tissue cushions that are painless. They arise above the dentate line.

Epidemiology

Tumors, pregnancy, portal hypertension, chronic cough (COPD), prostatic hyperplasia, or straining at stool or urine may precipitate the onset and/or thrombosis of hemorrhoids.

Management

Although most cases will **resolve spontaneously** within 2 weeks, **urgent hemorrhoidectomies** are generally recommended for thrombosed external hemorrhoids in patients with severe pain. Patients who choose medical management over surgery should take warm **sitz baths** (three times daily), receive **analgesics** and **stool softeners,** and **increase dietary fiber** intake. If medical treatment fails, symptoms recur, or complications arise (infection, bleeding), surgical treatment in the form of elastic band ligation, injection sclerotherapy, or excisional hemorrhoidectomy may be indicated.

Complications

Complications of surgery include incontinence, stricture formation, infections, and bleeding.

Breakout Point

> External hemorrhoids are painful; internal hemorrhoids are painless.

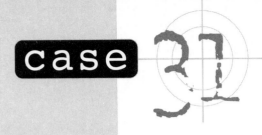

case

ID/CC	A 50-year-old construction worker complains of a **painful mass** in his **groin**.
HPI	The mass **enlarges with straining** and **disappears when he lies flat.**
PE	VS: normal. PE: barrel-shaped chest (due to COPD); abdomen soft, nontender, and nondistended; mass in inguinal region expands with coughing and diminishes with recumbency; when examining **finger is passed through scrotum into inguinal canal**, protrusion is felt on pad of finger.
Labs	Normal.
Imaging	**None.**

GENERAL SURGERY

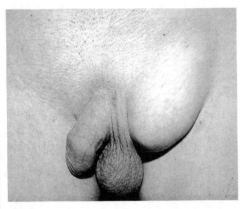

Figure 31-1. Presentation of patient showing large mass in groin.

case 31

Inguinal Hernia

Pathogenesis

A hernia is defined as a **protrusion of a viscus, or any part thereof,** through a **defect** in the **wall of the cavity** containing it. Inguinal hernias are classified as direct or indirect according to their anatomic relationship to the inferior epigastric vessels. **Indirect hernias** are due to **persistence of the processus vaginalis.** Herniation occurs **lateral** to the inferior epigastric artery, protrudes through the deep inguinal ring, and may extend into the scrotum. **Direct inguinal hernias** protrude through the floor of the inguinal canal (transversalis fascia and aponeurosis) through the Hesselbach triangle medial to the epigastric vessels. These are associated with tissue laxity (as in old age) and with any factor that **increases intra-abdominal pressure,** such as obesity, chronic cough, or straining with bowel movements or micturition (e.g., BPH).

Epidemiology

Inguinal hernias account for 75% of all hernias, are more common in males (versus femoral hernia), and are more commonly seen on the right side. **Indirect hernias are much more common** than direct hernias, particularly among children. Ten percent are bilateral.

Management

Acute incarceration or strangulation requires emergent surgical repair. In non-emergent cases, the patient is scheduled for **elective herniorrhaphy.**

Complications

Incarceration (irreducibility without vascular compromise), **strangulation** (ischemia and necrosis), perforated viscus, **intestinal obstruction** with fluid sequestration and electrolyte imbalance, and damage to the urinary bladder or spermatic cord during surgical repair.

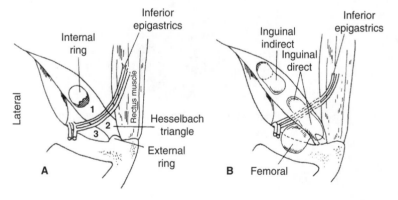

Figure 31-2. A. Hernias occur in Hesselbach triangle (2) inguinal canal (1, 2), and femoral space (3). **B.** Direct and indirect hernias occur above the inguinal ligament; femoral hernias occur below the inguinal ligament.

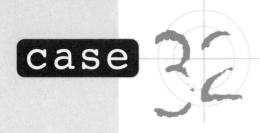

case 32

ID/CC	A 64-year-old insulin-dependent **diabetic** patient presents with a 4-month history of **dull, cramping** abdominal pain.
HPI	The pain generally begins an hour **after meals** (postprandial) and is epigastric in location. It lasts approximately 3 hours and has progressively been getting worse. The patient has a history of **atrial fibrillation** and **coronary artery disease**, with a **CABG** 6 months ago.
PE	HR 95, BP 140/90. Unremarkable abdominal exam, guaiac negative.
Labs	Labs WNL.
Imaging	KUB: unremarkable. Angiography showed arteriosclerotic stenoses of the proximal celiac and superior mesenteric arteries.

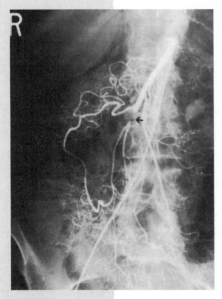

Figure 32-1. Superior mesenteric artery (SMA) embolism (*arrow*) with collateral circulation.

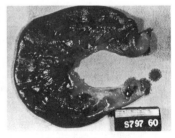

Figure 32-2. Nonocclusive vascular disease resulting in small bowel infarction.

case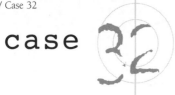

Mesenteric Ischemia

Pathogenesis

Mesenteric ischemia occurs due to a **reduction in intestinal blood** flow. The blood supply to the intestine is mainly through three gastrointestinal arteries: the **celiac axis, superior mesenteric artery (SMA),** and **inferior mesenteric artery (IMA).** There is significant collateral circulation to the intestine, which allows for partial protection from ischemia. Intestinal ischemia is divided into acute and chronic ischemia. Most cases are due to arterial causes. Acute mesenteric ischemia is due to sudden intestinal hypoperfusion. It is divided into **occlusive and nonocclusive obstruction of arterial or venous blood flow.** Occlusive arterial obstruction is most commonly due to emboli or thrombosis of mesenteric arteries (i.e., **atrial fibrillation).** Occlusive venous obstruction is most commonly due to thrombosis or segmental strangulation. Nonocclusive arterial hypoperfusion is mainly due to primary splanchnic vasoconstriction. Chronic mesenteric ischemia (also called intestinal angina) occurs due to **mesenteric atherosclerosis.**

Epidemiology

Mesenteric vascular disease occurs primarily in the **elderly** and is associated with extremely **high mortality** (approximately 80%).

Management

Intravenous fluid resuscitation, and nasogastric decompression if presence of ileus. Immediate surgical intervention for **resection of ischemic/necrotic bowel** if there are signs of peritonitis. Definitive treatment depends on the underlying etiology. An acute arterial thrombosis requires embolectomy, thrombolysis, or possibly surgical reconstruction (bypass surgery). Chronic mesenteric ischemia may require angioplasty, stenting, or surgical revascularization. Risk factor modification is important.

Complications

Sepsis/septic shock, multiple system organ failure, bowel necrosis/infarction, death.

Breakout Point

Mesenteric ischemia is associated with atrial fibrillation and mesenteric atherosclerosis.

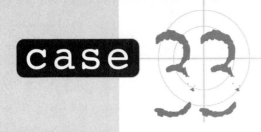

case 33

ID/CC   A 58-year-old man is evaluated for **yellowing of the skin and weight loss.**

HPI   Directed questioning reveals **dark urine** (CHOLURIA), **clay-colored stools** (ACHOLIA), and intense **pruritus.** He also has **anorexia** and a dull **abdominal pain.**

PE   VS: normal. PE: **emaciated** and markedly **jaundiced,** no abdominal tenderness or distention.

Labs   CBC: **low hemoglobin** (8.8 g/dL). ESR moderately elevated; **elevated glucose** (245 mg/dL). LFTs: **markedly elevated alkaline phosphatase; elevated total bilirubin** (12 mg/dL); **mildly elevated transaminases.** Hypercalcemia; amylase and lipase moderately elevated; elevated **serum CA 19-9** levels.

Imaging   See Figures 33-1 to 33-4.

GENERAL SURGERY

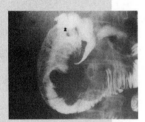

Figure 33-1. UGI. Displacement and narrowing of duodenal sweep due to mass effect of the head of the pancreas with ragged edges of infiltration.

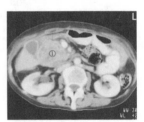

Figure 33-2. CT, abdomen. Heterogenous mass (*1*) in the pancreatic head.

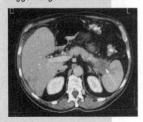

Figure 33-3. CT, abdomen. Another case—mass seen in pancreatic tail (*arrow*).

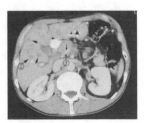

Figure 33-4. CT, abdomen. Another case—mass in pancreatic body (*1*).

case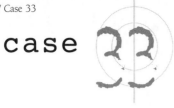

Pancreatic Cancer

Pathogenesis

The vast majority of pancreatic malignancies are **adeno-carcinomas,** two-thirds of which are ductal in origin and arise in the pancreatic head. Pancreatic carcinoma has been associated with a mutation in the *K-ras* onco-gene, Gardner syndrome, and colonic polyposis. It is also associated with **chronic pancreatitis** (calcific), **cigarette smoking, diabetes,** and hereditary mutations that are predisposing for pancreatic cancer.

Epidemiology

Pancreatic cancer is the fourth leading cause of cancer-related death in the United States. Only 15% to 20% of patients present with resectable disease. About 33,730 new cases will be diagnosed in 2007, with 32,300 expected deaths.

Management

Staging and diagnosis generally include some of the following imaging modalities: transcutaneous or endo-scopic ultrasound (US or EUS), computed tomography (CT), endoscopic retrograde cholangiopancreatogra-phy (ERCP), magnetic resonance imaging (MRI), and MR cholangiopancreatography (MRCP). Resectable (no portal or superior mesenteric artery, liver, or hepatic artery involvement) disease is treated by a **pancreaticoduodenectomy** (WHIPPLE PROCEDURE) fol-lowed by adjuvant chemotherapy and radiotherapy. Unresectable diseases are treated with definitive con-current chemoradiation.

Complications

Portal vein thrombosis, gastric outlet obstruction, metastatic disease, thromboembolic complications secondary to tumor-induced hypercoagulability, por-tal hypertension, splenomegaly, and jaundice.

Breakout Point

- Surgical treatment: WHIPPLE PROCEDURE.
- COURVOISIER SIGN: palpable and nontender gallbladder
- TROUSSEAU SYNDROME: migratory throm-bophlebitis

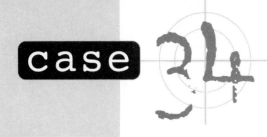
ID/CC An 18-year-old male **motorcyclist** was brought to the ED after colliding with an oncoming car. Paramedics found him **unresponsive and diaphoretic** with a **weak and rapid pulse**.

HPI After infusion of 2 L of Ringer lactate, he regained consciousness and complained of **severe left-sided abdominal pain** with **left thoracic pain on inspiration**. The abdominal pain **radiated to the upper posterior left back (scapula)**. He stabilized transiently but subsequently became increasingly hypotensive despite IVF resuscitation and transfusion of 2 units of red blood cells.

PE VS: T 95.6; **hypotension** (BP 75/40); **tachycardia** (HR 138). PE: alert and oriented; **skin cold and clammy** (hypovolemia); osseous crepitation (fracture) over left ribs 10 to 12; abdomen **distended;** ecchymosis and rebound tenderness in LUQ; diffuse guarding; palpable mass in LUQ (BALLANCE SIGN), scapular pain on elevation of foot of bed or on palpation of left subcostal region (KEHR SIGN).

Labs CBC: Hematocrit drop (25.0%); leukocytosis (17,500/mm³). LFTs: normal. Four-quadrant peritoneal tap reveals **gross blood.**

Imaging CXR: elevation of the left hemidiaphragm; medial displacement of gastric bubble, lateral fracture of left ribs 10 to 12; no hemopneumothorax. US/FAST: free fluid in all abdominal windows. CT: there is considerable blood in the perisplenic fossa as well as free blood in the peritoneal cavity around the liver (see Figure 34-1).

GENERAL SURGERY

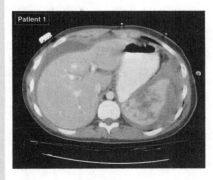

Figure 34-1.
Pathology in the spleen near the hilum. Considerable blood in the perisplenic fossa and in the peritoneal cavity around the liver.

case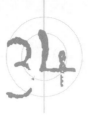

Splenic Rupture

Pathogenesis

The spleen is the **most commonly injured organ in blunt trauma.** Splenic injury is often an indicator of severe trauma, as 40% to 60% of splenic injuries present in association with other injuries. Because one-third of patients with a ruptured spleen do not initially present with frank hypotension and half may not have guarding and/or abdominal distention, a high index of suspicion must be maintained in trauma patients. There may be a **latent period** of up to 2 weeks between trauma and the onset of symptoms in some cases due to a capsular hematoma that liquefies over time. Although usually the result of blunt trauma **(including contact sports)**, splenic injury can also be secondary to penetrating trauma. **Lower rib fractures** are commonly associated with splenic rupture. Patients with **pathologic spleens** (due to hematologic disorders, infectious mononucleosis, malaria, leishmaniasis) are at higher risk.

Management

ACLS protocol: Airway, Breathing, Circulation, Disability, Exposure. Place **two large-bore IVs, start resuscitative fluids,** and insert a Foley catheter. Most EDs now use ultrasound **(focused abdominal sonography for trauma; FAST)** to test for free fluid in the abdomen, but a **diagnostic peritoneal lavage (DPL)** can also be used. A **negative lavage does not exclude** visceral damage. **Exploratory laparotomy** is indicated in the presence of positive DPL or FAST, free intraperitoneal air, peritoneal signs, inability to resuscitate, or recurring signs of shock despite aggressive resuscitation. If frank splenic rupture is found intra-operatively, a splenectomy is often required to stop hemorrhage. Nonoperative management may be indicated in hemodynamically stable patients.

Complications

Hemorrhagic shock, exsanguination. Post-splenectomy patients are at risk for infection by encapsulated bacteria and should receive prophylactic **pneumococcal and *Haemophilus influenzae* vaccinations.** Post-splenectomy sepsis occurs only rarely after post-traumatic splenectomy.

Breakout Point

> In blunt trauma, the spleen is the most commonly injured organ.

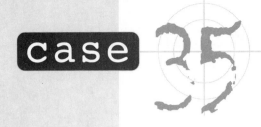

ID/CC	A **60-year-old man** complains of having **to wake up six to seven times at night to urinate** (NOCTURIA).
HPI	He also complains of urinary **urgency, weak stream, terminal dribbling,** and a need to strain in order to initiate micturition. He denies any weight loss, fatigue, or bone pain.
PE	VS: normal. PE: cardiopulmonary and abdominal exams normal; rectal exam reveals **enlarged, nontender prostate** gland that is **rubbery** throughout and without a palpable median ridge; 150 mL of **residual urine** obtained on postvoid catheterization.
Labs	UA: negative. CBC: normal. Alkaline and acid phosphatase normal; **PSA** 5.5 (normal of 5.4 based on gland size); BUN and creatinine normal.
Imaging	See Figure 35-1.

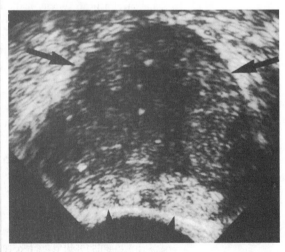

Figure 35-1. US, prostate. Transverse transrectal ultrasound scan shows enlarged **central transition zone** (*large arrows*) compressing peripheral zone (*small arrows*). (Posterior gland is in the lower part of the image.)

GENERAL SURGERY

case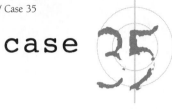

Benign Prostatic Hypertrophy

Pathogenesis

Benign prostatic hypertrophy (BPH) occurs as a result of **hyperplasia of stromal and epithelial tissue** in the peri-urethral zone of aging men. This testosterone-dependent hyperplasia may cause **urinary flow obstruction and/or obstructive prostatism.** The size of the gland on physical exam generally does not always correlate with symptoms. BPH usually originates in the periurethral and transition zones, while prostate cancer usually presents in the peripheral aspect of the prostate. It may coexist with carcinoma of the prostate, but **BPH is not considered a premalignant condition.** Note: Cold exposure, anticholinergic drugs, anesthetic agents, and alcohol may precipitate or worsen symptoms. BPH also increases PSA values, as does prostate cancer.

Epidemiology

The incidence of BPH increases with age; >90% of men have histologic evidence of BPH by age 85.

Management

Management is divided into medical and surgical therapies. Initial treatment is often medical with **5-α-reductase inhibitors** (e.g., finasteride) or **α-adrenergic blockers** (e.g., terazosin). **Surgery** may be done transurethrally (usually for glands <50 g), or the traditional open prostatectomy (retropubic, suprapubic, or perineal approach) may be performed. Transurethral resection of the prostate (**TURP**) is the most common procedure, with newer procedures including transurethral balloon dilatation (TUBD) and transurethral incision of the prostate (TUIP; most useful for subtrigonal obstruction).

Complications

Complications include **urinary tract infections** (from stagnant urine), bladder diverticula, calculi, hydronephrosis, and chronic pyelonephritis. Common surgical complications are sexual **impotence** (especially with the transperineal approach) and **retrograde ejaculation.**

Breakout Point

> Treatments for BPH are **5-α-reductase inhibitors,** **α-adrenergic blockers,** and **TURP.**

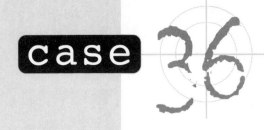
ID/CC A 32-year-old woman presents with a left breast lump on self-examination.

HPI The patient describes the lesion as firm and mobile. She is G2P2 and has **no family history** of breast cancer.

PE VS: stable. Breast exam: 1.5-cm rubbery, nontender nodule in the left lower outer quadrant. No nipple or skin changes; no axillary nodes.

Labs CBC: normal. Lytes: normal.

Imaging Mammography: **well-defined** mass with **sharply defined** margins.

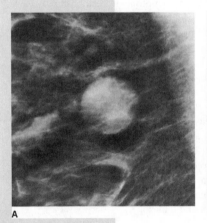 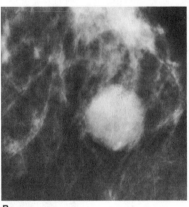

A   B

Figure 36-1. Round circumscribed mass with sharply defined margins on straight lateral **(A)** and craniocaudal **(B)** projections.

case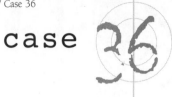

Benign Breast Nodule

Pathogenesis

Benign breast diseases include a number of conditions that can lead to clinical symptoms of **breast nodules, breast pain,** or **nipple discharge.** These diseases are generally related to hormonal and growth factors that regulate the breast tissue.

Epidemiology

Benign breast diseases are very common. For example, fibrocystic changes occur in 60% of premenopausal woman. Common causes for breast mass are fibroadenoma (this case) and cysts. Fibrocystic disease, mastitis, large pendulous breast, and hidradenitis suppurativa can all cause breast pain. Infections and cysts can cause nipple discharge. Bloody discharge generally indicates cancer.

Management

History should include symptoms in relationship to menstrual cycles, the color and location of nipple discharge, hormone use, and prior treatments. Risk factors for breast cancer should also be identified. Physical exam should aim to differentiate between benign lesions and malignant lesions. Breast cancers tend to be immobile, nontender, with irregular border and occasional skin dimpling. **Mammography** is the diagnostic imaging modality of choice, and **breast ultrasound** is used to assess cysts. Almost all solid lesions are biopsied to rule out breast cancer. Proliferative lesions that may lead to breast cancer should be followed closely. Once the breast condition is diagnosed as benign, the goal of therapy is symptomatic relief. Medical management includes hormone therapies such as tamoxifen and danazol.

Complications

Pain, infection, and breast cancer.

Breakout Point

- Smooth, well-demarcated lumps usually benign
- Characteristics of breast cancer on mammography:
  Increased density
  Irregular margins
  Spiculation
  Clustered irregular microcalcifications

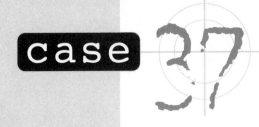

case 37

ID/CC A 55-year-old woman presents with a right breast **nodule**.

HPI The patient felt a small nodule in the right breast on self-examination. She has had yearly mammography screening, and no history of mammography abnormalities. She is G0P0 (**NULLIPARITY**). Her menarche was at 8 (**early menarche**), and she is still premenopausal (**late menopause**). She has no **family history** of breast cancer.

PE VS: afebrile. Breast exam: 1- to 2-cm nodule in the right upper outer quadrant. No cervical, supraclavicular, or axillary lymphadenopathy.

Labs CBC: normal. Lytes: normal.

Imaging Mammography: an **irregular** mass with a **spiculated** margin in the right upper outer quadrant that was not present on previous mammograms.

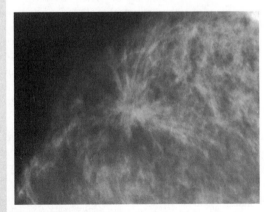

Figure 37-1. Breast US. 1.5-cm hypoechoic mass in the right upper outer quadrant.

case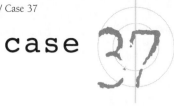

Breast Cancer

Pathogenesis

Risk factors for breast cancer include increased **estrogen exposure (early menarche, late menopause, nulliparity, and hormone replacement), family history, genetic mutations (BRCA-1, BRCA-2), ionizing radiation at young age,** dietary/environmental factors, and premalignant lesions. Breast cancer can evolve from the ductal cells or the lobular cells in the breast. In situ carcinomas include ductal carcinoma in situ (DCIS) and lobular carcinoma in situ (LCIS). Invasive carcinomas include invasive ductal carcinoma (76%), invasive lobular carcinoma (8%), and uncommon types such as mucinous carcinoma or tubular carcinoma.

Epidemiology

Breast cancer is the **most common female cancer** and the **second most common cause of cancer death in women** in the United States. An estimated 212,920 American women will be diagnosed with breast cancer and 40,970 women will have died from this disease in 2007.

Management

Curative treatment modalities include **mastectomy (less common)** or **breast-conserving surgery (lumpectomy) and adjuvant radiation.** Early invasive cancers are treated with surgical resection (mastectomy or lumpectomy) with **sentinel node biopsy.** Patients at risk for systemic disease will receive chemotherapy, and patients undergoing breast-conserving surgery will receive adjuvant radiation. Patients with high-risk/advanced disease will be treated with combined-modality therapy with surgery, chemotherapy, and radiotherapy.

Complications

Locally advanced disease can lead to skin erosion and brachioplexus invasion, causing severe pain. Metastatic disease to bone, brain, and lung can lead to pain, neurologic symptoms, and death.

Breakout Point

- Mammography screening should start at age 40 for average-risk patients. Patients with a higher-than-average risk for breast cancer should begin screening at an earlier age, and MRI may be helpful.
- Patients with either **BRCA-1** or **BRCA-2** mutation are also at high risk to develop **ovarian cancer.**

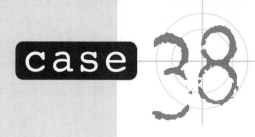

ID/CC   A 28-year-old woman comes to the ER for severe abdominal pain, with nausea and vomiting.

HPI   On your review of systems, she reports many **years** of **intermittent crampy abdominal pain, diarrhea,** and recent **weight loss.** She also reports that her mother has always had GI problems (**family history**).

PE   VS: temp **38.3°C**, otherwise normal. PE: general-**thin, mild pallor;** abdominal-diffuse **tenderness;** rectal-**skin tags,** no frank blood, but **guaiac positive** on digital exam.

Labs   CBC: **Hb 11, Hct 33.5**; otherwise normal. (−) **p-ANCA** and (+) **ASCA.**

Imaging   Colonoscopy: **cobblestone** appearance and **skip lesions,** narrowing of the terminal ileum lumen with nodularity and ulcerations. Small-bowel follow-through series: narrowing of the terminal ileum and right colon.

Pathology   Focal ulcerations with both acute and chronic inflammation.

GENERAL SURGERY

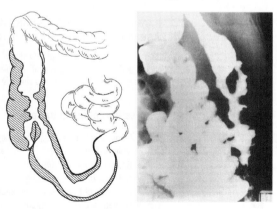

Figure 38-1. Small bowel follow through series showing pathology in the ileal cecal valve and right colon.

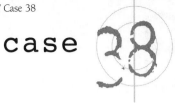

case 38

Crohn Disease

Pathogenesis

Although the cause of Crohn disease remains unclear, it manifests as **transmural inflammation leading to the formation of ulcers, fistulas, fibrosis, perforations, and obstruction throughout the entire GI tract from mouth to anus.** Risk factors include family history, smoking, and nutritional deficiencies (Zn).

Epidemiology

The incidence of Crohn disease in the United States is 6 to 7.1:100,000. The peak incidence occurs between the ages of 15 and 30 years. It is impossible to distinguish Crohn and UC in up to 15% of patients with IBS.

Management

Diagnostic workup is similar to workup for ulcerative colitis: serum autoantibody tests, colonoscopy, and biopsy. Medical management includes oral **5-ASA agents, antibiotics, and corticosteroids.** Anti-diarrheal therapy should also be initiated. In obstructed patients, conservative therapy with NPO, NG tube suction, IV fluids, and pain control will usually lead to resolution. For refractory patients, **azathioprine** and **6-MP** can be tried, as well as **methotrexate** and **infliximab (Remicade)** for severe cases. Surgery is not always recommended primarily because of high likelihood of disease recurrence, though it should be undertaken for abscesses, strictures, and fistulas as appropriate.

Complications

Malabsorption, diarrhea, obstruction, hemorrhage, perforation, fistulas, abcesses, toxic megacolon. Crohn disease can also cause extra abdominal symptoms including uveitis, erythema nodosum, cholangitis, and arthritis.

▓ **TABLE 38-1 AREAS OF INVOLVEMENT: CROHN DISEASE VERSUS ULCERATIVE COLITIS**

Crohn	Ulcerative Colitis
Entire GI tract	Largely limited to rectum and colon
Skip lesions	Continuous involvement

Breakout Point

Features of Crohn Disease

- Involvement of the small bowel (which excludes ulcerative colitis)
- Sparing of the rectum
- Absence of gross bleeding
- Presence of bothersome perianal disease
- Focality of gross and microscopic lesions, the presence of granulomas, or the occurrence of fistulae
- Skip lesions

Antibodies to distinguish Crohn from UC: neg p-ANCA and pos ASCA = Crohn disease

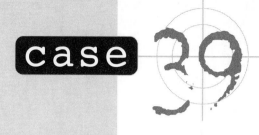

case 29

ID/CC A 29-year-old female presents with **diarrhea** and recurrent **rectal bleeding** and **passage of mucus** over the past 3 weeks.

HPI She reports feeling **weak** but has had no recent fevers or illnesses. She also denies any past medical history but says that her brother has a type of inflammatory bowel syndrome **(family history)**.

PE VS: normal. PE: general—**thin, pallor;** abdominal—soft, **tender in left lower quadrant;** rectal—**tenderness** on digital exam, **red blood** on glove.

Labs CBC: **Hb 9.6, Hct 28.5.** Otherwise normal. Flexible sigmoidoscopy: erythematous, edematous, easily friable mucosa, and continuous ulcerations along the intestinal walls.

Imaging Extensive pseudopolyposis with foreshortening of the bowel.

Pathology Biopsy reveals inflammation limited to the mucosal layer of the colon, crypt abscesses, and loss of mucin in goblet cells.

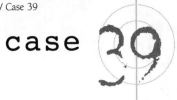

case

Ulcerative Colitis

Pathogenesis Full understanding of the causes of ulcerative colitis remains elusive, though it is known that the disease causes recurrent inflammation of the mucosal layers of the intestines, largely limited to the colon. Risk factors include genetic factors (family history), oral contraceptives, and infectious agents.

Epidemiology The incidence and prevalence rates are 3 to 15 per 100,000 and 50 to 80 per 100,000, respectively.

Management Diagnostic workup generally includes flexible sigmoidoscopy, barium enema, and ultrasonography. Acute bleeding should be managed as other lower GI bleeds with fluid resuscitation, etc. Long-term management depends on the extent of the disease, which is largely based on the total area of involvement from the rectum. Therapy begins with **5-ASA suppositories** (most effective) and **steroid foams.** If there is no response or topical therapy is not tolerated, **oral sulfasalazine** and **5-ASA** is the next step. **Limited courses of oral prednisone** should also be considered in nonresponders but has more systemic side effects. Supplemental **iron** and **antibiotics** should be started on a PRN basis, as well as **antidiarrheal** agents (but should not be used in acute flares because they may precipitate toxic megacolon). Severe cases require bowel rest and **IV steroids, cyclosporine, azathioprine,** or **6-MP.** Massive hemorrhage, toxic megacolon, and disease refractory to medical therapy require surgery. In an emergency, **abdominal colectomy with ileostomy and Hartmann closure** is preferred, while more elective cases allow choices as to the extent of **proctocolectomy, type of ileostomy, and later anastamosis.**

Complications Diarrhea, hemorrhage, anemia, perforation, colonic stricture, **sclerosing cholangitis, toxic megacolon, colon cancer (increased risk).**

■ TABLE 39-1 CROHN DISEASE VERSUS ULCERATIVE COLITIS

	Crohn Disease	Ulcerative Colitis
Small-Bowel Involvement	Common	Never
Colon Involvement	Common	Always
Rectal Involvement	Rare	Common
Anal Involvement	Common	Rare
Extent of Disease	Patchy	Continuous
Depth of Involvement	Deep	Superficial
Fistula Formation	Common	Rare
Strictures and Stenosis	Common	Rare
Granuloma	Common	Rare
Surgical Treatment	Resection of the affected bowel	Usually total colectomy

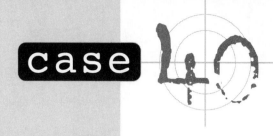

case 40

ID/CC 40-year-old **obese** male presents with **daytime sleepiness** (SOMNOLENCE).

HPI Directed questioning reveals **hypnagogic hallucinations** and nightmares. His wife reports that he **snores heavily** with periods of silence **(apnea)** at night. The patient naps 4 times per day but never feels refreshed. He has fallen asleep while driving on two occasions. He denies cataplexy or sleep paralysis.

PE VS: **hypertension** (BP 150/90). PE: **obese** (260 lb); nasal voice; **retrognathia; oropharynx narrowed** by excessive soft tissue; large tonsils; pendulous uvula and prominent tongue (MACROGLOSSIA); large neck.

Labs TFTs normal. **Polysomnography** reveals 20 apneic spells/hr (**>5 apneas/hr** is diagnostic) lasting 20 to 30 seconds each, with O_2 saturation dropping to as low as 80% during episodes.

Imaging CXR: large pulmonary arteries and redistribution of pulmonary blood flow.

case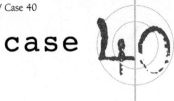

Obstructive Sleep Apnea

Pathogenesis

Relaxation during sleep can cause airway collapse and obstruction with resulting apnea in patients with structural narrowing of the upper airway. Inspiratory effort is present but unsuccessful.

Epidemiology

Most commonly affects **middle-aged obese males.** Other causes of **anatomic narrowing** of the upper airways (e.g., tonsillar hypertrophy, macroglossia, micrognathia) also predispose.

Management

Weight reduction and avoidance of alcohol/sedative medications at night are first-line approaches. The most effective therapy is **continuous positive airway pressure (CPAP)** at night. Mechanical prostheses can also be considered. Refractory cases may require surgical treatment, such as uvulopalatopharyngoplasty, septoplasty, adenotonsillectomy, and/or mandibular advancement to improve tolerance of CPAP. If these measures fail, tracheostomy is considered.

Complications

Complications include systemic hypertension, ischemic heart disease, pulmonary hypertension, cor pulmonale, and respiratory failure. Sleep apnea patients may be especially sensitive to narcotics due to compromised respiratory drive at baseline. Unexpected death during sleep may result from MI, arrhythmias, and asphyxia.

Breakout Point

- Most common in obese middle-aged males
- Results from upper airway obstruction
- Treated with weight reduction, avoiding alcohol/sedation before bed, CPAP, and possibly surgery to decrease upper airway obstruction

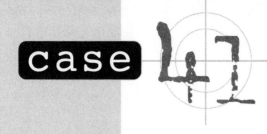

case 47

ID/CC   A 38-year-old male comes to the clinic for his **third visit** in 2 months complaining of continued **epigastric pain, nausea,** and acid **reflux symptoms** (burning in substernal chest, worst after eating).

HPI   He reports that he has been taking his **H₂-antagonist** as prescribed and that he finished the entire course of *Helicobacter pylori* **treatment** (2 weeks) **without major improvement** in symptoms. He also complains of sporadic episodes of **diarrhea.**

PE   VS: normal. PE: general—**thin;** abdominal—moderate tenderness in epigastric area.

Labs   **Fasting serum gastrin** concentration 220 pg/mL (normal <110 pg/mL).

Imaging **Octreoscan:** two pancreatic nodules around 2 cm in size.

case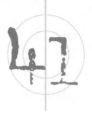

Zollinger-Ellison Syndrome

Pathogenesis

Gastrinomas arise from endodermal stem cells and primarily form in the duodenum (70%) and pancreas. Extreme levels of gastrin act with a direct trophic effect on parietal cells and cause release of histamine, both of which increase acid production. Metastatic disease is present in up to one-third of cases of patients with gastrin, with the liver being the most common site of spread.

Epidemiology

Estimated incidence of Zollinger-Ellison syndrome ranges from 0.1% to 1% of patients with peptic ulcer disease. Patients are normally diagnosed between the ages of 18 and 50 with a male/female ratio of approximately 1.5:1. Gastrinomas can occur sporadically but often appear as part of multiple endocrine neoplasia type 1 (MEN I).

Management

Diagnostic studies include **fasting serum gastrin** concentration, which should not exceed the normal upper limit of 110 pg/mL. The **secretin stimulation test** should also be performed, as it allows the differentiation of gastrinomas from other causes of hypergastrinemia. Secretin stimulates a release of gastrin by gastrinoma cells but inhibits the release of gastrin by normal gastric G-cells. **Somatostatin receptor imaging with Octreoscan and SPECT** can help localize tumor. **Endoscopic ultrasound** can also be used to image tumors for needle biopsy and pathologic analysis. Medical management includes high-dose **proton-pump inhibitors**. In those without evidence of metastases or MEN I, **laparotomy** can be performed to remove the gastrinoma and explore for metastatic disease. **Intraoperative transillumination** is useful for detecting very small gastrinomas. Treatment of **metastatic disease** is much more difficult and offers limited benefit.

Complications

Peptic ulcer disease (90% of patients with ZE) resistant to medical treatment, diarrhea/steatorrhea, metastatic disease, other manifestations of MEN I (parathyroid, pituitary, and pancreatic islet cell tumors).

Breakout Point

Dx and Rx of Zollinger–Ellison
• Dx—fasting serum gastrin
• Dx—secretin stimulation
• Rx—proton-pump inhibitors
• Rx—surgery for sporadic tumors
• Rx—chemotherapy for metastases

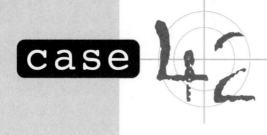
ID/CC A 5-year-old boy presents with several episodes of passing **dark red bloody stool.**

HPI The patient reports occasional maroon-colored stool for the **last month.** He denies pain or any other associated symptoms, and has no other known medical history.

PE Abdominal exam is negative, guaiac positive. No signs of an acute abdomen.

Labs CBC: normal WBC, Hb 9 (anemia), Plt 150. Coagulation studies were normal.

Imaging KUB: normal. CT of the abdomen and pelvis: normal. **Technetium Tc-99m scintiscan** is positive.

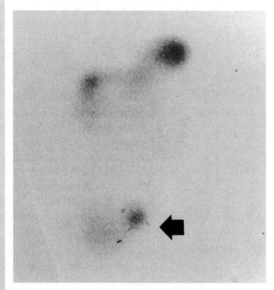

Figure 42-1. Tissue resembles gastric mucosa.

GENERAL SURGERY

case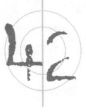

Meckel Diverticulum

Pathogenesis

Meckel diverticulum is the **most common congenital abnormality** of the digestive tract. It is a **persistent vitelline duct** (omphalomesenteric duct). It occurs on the antimesenteric border of the ileum, usually **2 feet proximal to the ileocecal valve**. On average, the diverticulum is **2 inches long** and is a **true diverticulum**. The heterotopic mucosa is most often gastric in origin, which can cause peptic ulceration and lead to pain, bleeding, and perforation. Hemorrhage occurs almost exclusively before age 10. In older patients, Meckel diverticulum is usually an incidental finding—most patients are asymptomatic. Clinical presentation varies and includes gastrointestinal bleeding, intestinal obstruction, and inflammation of the diverticulum. Meckel diverticulitis may present as acute abdomen. Technetium-99m (99mTc) pertechnetate scan is the imaging modality of choice to diagnose Meckel diverticula. The scan detects gastric mucosa, as approximately 50% of Meckel diverticula have ectopic gastric cells. Other tests such as colonoscopy and angiography can help in determining the location of bleeding.

Epidemiology

Meckel diverticulum occurs in 2% of the population.

Management

Symptomatic patients are usually acutely ill, and require intravenous fluids and NPO status. Broad-spectrum antibiotic therapy should be started in cases of acute Meckel diverticulitis, strangulation, perforation, or signs of sepsis. With significant bleeding, a blood transfusion may be necessary. Patients with bowel obstruction may require nasogastric decompression. The definitive treatment of a Meckel diverticulum is excision of the diverticulum along with the adjacent ileal segment.

Complications

Abdominal pain, bowel obstruction, hemorrhage, diverticulitis, umbilical fistula, other umbilical lesions, and intussusception.

Breakout Point

Rule of 2's
2 percent (of the population), **2** feet (from the ileocecal valve), **2** inches (in length), only **2%** are symptomatic

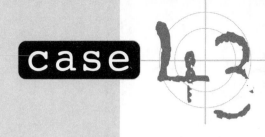
case 43

ID/CC A 28-year-old male construction worker complains of **severe leg pain** after an 80-pound concrete beam fell onto his left leg.

HPI The injury was confined to his left leg with the limb trapped under the beam for 30 minutes before help arrived. In the ED, x-rays revealed **no fracture** and he was diagnosed with **soft-tissue crush injury.** Six hours later he complains of **worsening pain** in the leg and new **numbness** over the top of the foot.

PE Afebrile, HR 95, BP: 135/85. Patient uncomfortable and restless. Left leg with extensive swelling and bruising (ECCHYMOSIS). Soft-tissue compartments are **rock hard** and **painful** with palpation. Unable to actively dorsiflex the great toe or ankle. Exquisite pain with **passive** range of motion of the toes. Sensation to light touch absent over dorsum of the foot including the first web space. Decreased DP and PT pulses.

Labs CBC/Chemistries: normal.

Imaging None indicated.

case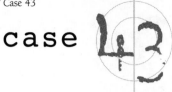

Compartment Syndrome

Pathogenesis

Compartment syndrome occurs when pressure builds up in a confined space within the body, which can lead to **capillary vessel collapse, decreased venous return, tissue ischemia,** and **necrosis.** Pressure buildup occurs secondary to swelling of the tissues or accumulation of fluid within a compartment. If pressure remains elevated for extended periods of time, muscle and nerve function is compromised and **permanent tissue necrosis can occur.** Compartment syndrome occurs most commonly in the muscle compartments of the lower leg and forearm but can also occur in the thigh, hand, foot, and other locations. Injuries that lead to compartment syndrome often involve extensive soft-tissue damage (crush injury, gunshot wound, compound fracture); however, compartment syndrome can also occur after prolonged limb compression, postoperatively, after accidental infusions of saline or other chemicals into soft tissue, or in rare cases, after prolonged exercise.

Management

Patients with high risk for compartment syndrome should be managed with ice, strict elevation, and serial physical exams. In some cases, serial quantitative compartment pressure checks may also be required. Compartment pressures can be measured directly using a variety of commercially available catheter devices. Normal compartment pressure is <10 mm Hg. True compartment syndrome is an indication for emergent surgery to **release the involved compartments** (FASCIOTOMY) and return capillary blood flow to tissues. Due to the extent of swelling, the overlying skin is often left open after fasciotomy and many patients will require later surgeries for wound closure or skin grafting. Depending on the extent of damage at the time of diagnosis, the effects of increased compartment pressures can be reversible. Permanent muscle and nerve damage with resultant loss of function and scarring leads to a volkmann contracture of the limb.

Complications

Muscle necrosis, permanent nerve damage, limb ischemia (Volkmann contracture), and reperfusion syndrome.

Breakout Point

6 P's:
Pain, Pallor, Pulse lessness, Paralysis, Paresthesia, Poikilethermia

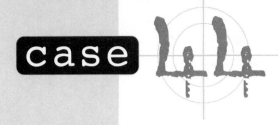

case 44

ID/CC	A **70-year-old** man presents with **fresh blood in the urine** without pain (PAINLESS HEMATURIA).
HPI	The patient has a 60-pack-year **smoking** history.
PE	VS: normal. PE: benign.
Labs	CBC: normal. Calcium and alkaline phosphatase normal. UA: 500 RBCs/HPF.
Imaging	**Cystoscopy:** 2-cm mass at the right ureteral orifice. CT of the abdomen and pelvis: see Figure 44-1.

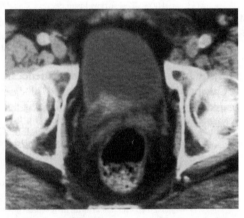

Figure 44-1. CT of the abdomen and pelvis. Mass at the right ureteral orifice. There is ureteral dilation, which may be partially mechanical.

GENITOURINARY

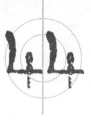

case

Bladder Cancer

Pathogenesis

More than **90% of bladder cancers are transitional-cell carcinomas.** Tumors are classified by grade and growth patterns. Risk factors include exposure to industrial solvents and dyes, **cigarette smoking,** chronic *Schistosoma hematobium* infection (squamous cell cancer), and past exposure to radiation or cyclophophamide. The most common presenting symptoms are intermittent painless hematuria and voiding symptoms (urgency, frequency).

Epidemiology

Bladder cancer is the **fourth** most common cancer in men and the tenth in women. Male-to-female ratio is 2.7:1, with those affected usually between the ages of 50 and 70. Superficial bladder cancer has an excellent prognosis, with 5-year survival rates of 82% to 100%. The survival rate decreases as depth of invasion increases.

Management

Diagnostic workup generally includes **urinalysis, urine cytology,** and cystoscopy. **Cystoscopy** is the main diagnostic and staging modality for bladder cancer. Radiographic evaluation can include CT, MRI, ultrasound, and intravenous pyelogram (IVP). IVP is especially helpful in diagnosing or ruling out urothelial cancers (ureter). Treatment depends on the stage of the tumor. **TURBT** and periodic follow-up with cystoscopy and biopsy are appropriate for low-grade superficial lesions. Intravesical chemotherapy or Bacillus Calmette-Guérin (BCG) immunotherapy can reduce the risk of recurrence after resection. **Muscle invasive disease** (T2 and higher) has a high risk for metastases. These can be treated with either TURBT followed by chemotherapy and radiotherapy, or partial/radical cystectomy with lymph node dissection in combination with radiation and/or chemotherapy. The small bowel may be used to create a continent reservoir for urine (KOCH POUCH).

Complications

Ileus, bowel obstruction, enterocutaneous fistula, rectal injury, and electrolyte abnormalities after Koch pouch.

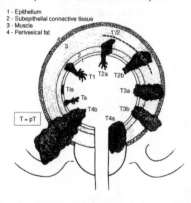

1 - Epithelium
2 - Subepithelial connective tissue
3 - Muscle
4 - Perivesical fat

Figure 44-2. Local tumor (T) staging of bladder cancer.

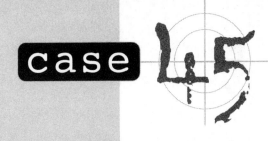

case 45

ID/CC	A **60-year-old man** presents with **elevated PSA** of 5.8.
HPI	He has had PSA screening since age 50. His PSA value has been gradually **rising** over the years. His PSA value 1 year ago was 4.8.
PE	VS: normal. PE: abdominal and lung exam normal; testes normal; digital rectal exam (DRE) reveals normal sphincter tone and a diffusely enlarged prostate gland with a **painless, hard nodule** in the left base.
Labs	CBC: normal. Electrolytes normal.
Imaging	CT, pelvis: no lymphadenopathy. Endorectal coil MRI: no extracapsular extension.
Pathology	**Gleason** $3 + 3 = 6$ **adenocarcinoma** in 3/12 cores.

case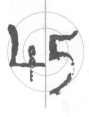

Prostate Cancer

Pathogenesis

Almost all prostate cancers are adenocarcinomas and are testosterone sensitive. Risk factors include older age, race (more common in African-Americans), diet, and chronic prostatitis.

Epidemiology

Prostate cancer is the **most common cancer in American men** (except for non-melanoma skin cancer). It is estimated that 234,460 men will be diagnosed in 2007 and 27,350 will die of the disease.

Management

Prostate cancer screening should be initiated at age 50. Screening exams include **DRE** and **PSA** (controversial). Diagnosis is based on perineal/transrectal ultrasound-guided biopsy (usually 12 or more cores). Clinical staging workup includes DRE, CT of the abdomen/pelvis and/or endorectal coil MRI to rule out lymph node metastases, extracapsular extension and seminal vesicle invasion. High-risk patients may need **bone scan** to rule out systemic disease. Low-risk prostate cancer can be managed by **radical prostatectomy** (open, laparoscopic, robotic), **brachytherapy** (radioactive seeds), **external beam radiotherapy,** or **active surveillance** (watchful waiting). Intermediate-risk prostate cancer can be treated with radical prostatectomy, brachytherapy, or external beam radiotherapy combined with **androgen deprivation.** Surgery for intermediate-risk prostate cancer is associated with higher rate of PSA recurrence, and may need adjuvant or salvage radiotherapy. High-risk prostate cancer can be managed by androgen deprivation and external beam radiotherapy, or androgen deprivation alone. Metastatic prostate cancer is treated with androgen deprivation; chemotherapy has not been very effective in prostate cancer treatment.

Complications

Urinary obstruction, metastatic disease leading to pain and death. Treatment morbidities include impotency (surgery and radiotherapy), rectal bleeding (radiotherapy), and urinary incontinence (surgery).

Breakout Point

Gleason Score

The Gleason grading system is based on architectural features of prostate cancer. Tumors are graded from 1 to 5, based on the growth pattern and degree of differentiation, with grade 1 being the most and grade 5 the least differentiated. The composite Gleason score is then derived by adding the two most prevalent differentiation patterns (a primary grade and a secondary grade). It is important to know that a score of 3 + 4 is better than 4 + 3 even though both composite scores are 7.

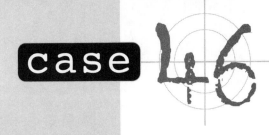

case 46

ID/CC	A 50-year-old **white male** presents with **blood in the urine** (hematuria).
HPI	He has a 40-pack-year **smoking** history. He denies any fever or chills.
PE	VS: Afebrile. PE: alert; no jaundice; no cyanosis; lungs clear to auscultation; no costovertebral angle tenderness.
Labs	CBC: **Hb 17.4 g/dL** (due to erythropoietin secreted by tumor; advanced disease may present with anemia). UA: **hematuria.**
Imaging	Renal US: a large mass in the left kidney.

case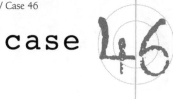

Renal Cell Carcinoma

Pathogenesis

Renal cell carcinoma (RCC) accounts for 85% of renal parenchymal cancers and classically presents with **hematuria, flank pain,** and **palpable mass.** Patients frequently present with **painless hematuria** (gross or microscopic), pathologic fracture, skin nodules, or left varicocele (tumor extension to left renal artery). RCC is associated with **cigarette smoking,** obesity, hypertension, and **von Hippel-Lindau (VHL)** disease, as well as acquired cystic kidney disease associated with end-stage renal disease. **Paraneoplastic syndromes** include anemia, hepatic dysfunction, fever, hypercalcemia, cachexia, and **erythrocytosis** (secondary to elevated erythropoietin levels).

Epidemiology

An estimated of 39,000 people will be diagnosed with RCC and almost 13,000 will die from RCC in the United States in 2007. RCC occurs predominantly in the **sixth to eighth decade** of life. More cases are diagnosed incidentally on abdominal CT.

Management

CT scan is diagnostic and is the staging procedure of choice. Surgical resection is the primary and curative treatment for renal cancer. Early-stage disease is treated with **radical nephrectomy** (adrenal, local nodes, distal ureter). Advanced disease can be treated with surgical resection followed by chemotherapy and immunotherapy.

Complications

Intratumoral bleeding, leg edema, and **varicocele** due to vena cava thrombosis; high-output cardiac failure (AV shunting); pulmonary embolism, renal colic due to clots, polycythemia, metastatic disease (lungs, bone), paraneoplastic syndromes (e.g., hypercalcemia), obstructive uropathy, and **pathologic fractures.**

Breakout Point

Von Hippel-Lindau Disease

An inherited, autosomal-dominant syndrome that is associated with hemangioblastomas, clear cell RCCs, pheochromocytomas, endolymphatic sac tumors of the middle ear, serous cystadenomas and neuroendocrine tumors of the pancreas, and papillary cystadenomas of the epididymis and broad ligament

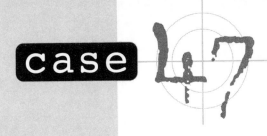

case **47**

ID/CC A 28-year-old man presents with a **painless enlargement of his testes** of several months' duration.

HPI The patient was initially unconcerned because the enlargement was painless. He has become more concerned because of continued growth and an increased sensation of heaviness. He reveals that he was diagnosed with **cryptorchidism** in the right testicle as an infant; the condition was corrected by orchiopexy at age 1.

PE VS: normal. PE: in no acute distress; lung and abdominal exams normal; diffuse enlargement of testes noted on GU exam; rectal exam unremarkable.

Labs CBC: normal. **Mildly elevated hCG;** normal α-fetoprotein.

Imaging **Scrotal US:** intratesticular hypoechoic mass. CXR/CT, abdomen and pelvis (to look for metastases): normal.

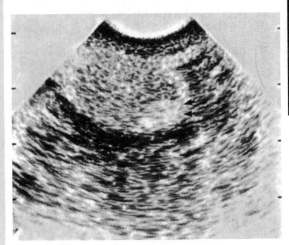

Figure 47-1. Lesion located on the posterior aspect replacing over half of the testis.

GENITOURINARY

case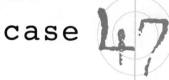

Testicular Cancer

Pathogenesis

Testicular germ-cell tumors are classified as **seminomas** (40% of cases) and **nonseminomatous germ-cell tumors** (embryonal-cell carcinomas, teratomas, choriocarcinomas, and mixed-cell types). Non-germ-cell tumors (Leydig cell, Sertoli cell, gonadoblastoma) comprise the remaining 5% to 10%. Risk factors include cryptorchidism, prior history of testicular cancer, family history, HIV infection, in utero exposure to estrogen, and androgen insensitivity syndromes.

Epidemiology

Testicular cancer is the most common solid malignancy affecting males between the ages of 15 and 35.

Management

Workup includes serum marker studies, scrotal ultrasound, and abdominal/pelvic CT (rule out lymph node metastases). PET/CT may be helpful. **Inguinal orchiectomy** is both a diagnostic and a treatment procedure. Stages I and nonbulky II seminomas are generally treated with adjuvant **retroperitoneal irradiation** or **watchful waiting.** Advanced-stage disease is treated with adjuvant **chemotherapy.**

Complications

Testicular tumors may be complicated by metastases to the retroperitoneum (low back pain), lungs (cough), or vena cava (lower extremity edema), or they may lead to intratesticular hemorrhage.

Breakout Point

> Testicular cancer is one of the most curable solid neoplasms, with more than a 90% cure rate.

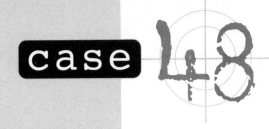

case 48

ID/CC	A **16-year-old** male presents with an **acute onset** of left **groin swelling** and **pain.** The pain is **sharp, intermittently worse,** with associated **nausea and vomiting.**
HPI	This pain began shortly after a flag football game (i.e., vigorous physical activity). He has had a similar but less severe pain intermittently, which resolved on its own.
PE	VS: normal. PE: **tender, edematous** left testicle in **transverse lie,** with **absent cremasteric reflex** on ipsilateral side. Check for signs of alternative diagnoses, such as penile discharge (STDs), abdominal pain (hernia, appendicitis), flank pain (kidney stone), etc.
Labs	Not relevant.
Imaging	**Color Doppler ultrasonography** is used to evaluate blood flow to the testicle.

case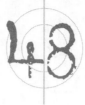

Testicular Torsion

Pathogenesis

Congenital abnormalities in the fixation of the testis to the tunica vaginalis can allow the gonad to torse on the spermatic cord, resulting in ischemia from arterial insufficiency and venous outflow obstruction.

Epidemiology

Testicular torsion is the most acute and potentially serious of all presentations of the acute scrotum. It most often happens in neonates and in males near the age of puberty, but can occur at any age. The differential diagnosis must also include **epididymitis** (fever, dysuria, and slower onset of pain) and **torsion of the appendix testis** (intact cremasteric reflex).

Management

If the clinical presentation is appropriate and suspicion high, then **immediate surgical exploration** is required, as waiting for an ultrasound may result in more ischemic time and ultimately contribute to orchiectomy. Fixation of **both** testicles is required after detorsion, as the fixation defect is likely bilateral. If surgery is not possible, then **manual detorsion** may be attempted by turning the affected testicle laterally. Successful manual detorsion will result in relief of pain and a lower, more vertical position of the testicle. However, surgical exploration is **still mandatory** to fixate the testicles and ensure that there is no residual torsion.

Complications

Recurrence, infection, and loss of testicle.

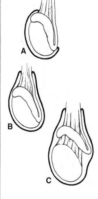

Figure 48-1. Anatomy of testicular torsion.
A. Normal anatomy. **B.** Bell-clapper deformity, allowing torsion of both epididymis and testicle.
C. Variant anatomy, allowing torsion below the epididymis.

Breakout Point

Presenting Symptoms of Testicular Torsion	
• Tender	• Transverse lie
• Edematous	• Absent cremaster reflex

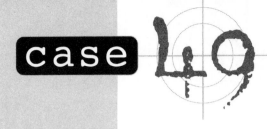

case **49**

ID/CC   A 40-year-old woman presents with right shoulder pain after **falling backward and sideways onto her outstretched hand** (forced abduction and external rotation).

HPI   She noticed **deformity** of her shoulder immediately after the fall. She presents clutching her right arm to her body and is in extreme pain.

PE   VS: normal. PE: loss of round shoulder contour; a **depression** is easily palpable under the acromion (sulcus sign); humeral head palpable through axilla; any attempts at range-of-motion testing of the shoulder are met with mechanical resistance and cause significant pain; normal sensation over deltoid and active firing of deltoid (no evidence of axillary nerve palsy); fully neurovascularly intact to the hand.

Labs   CBC: normal.

Imaging   XR, right shoulder (AP, oblique, axillary views): **humeral head dislocated anteriorly** and displaced to the **subcoracoid** position.

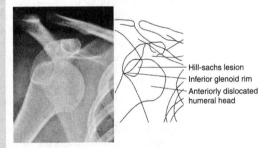

Figure 49-1. Anterior shoulder dislocation. Anteroposterior film of the shoulder shows the typical appearance of anterior dislocation. The humeral head lies beneath the inferior rim of the glenoid.

ORTHOPEDIC

case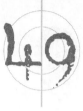

Shoulder Dislocation

Pathogenesis

The glenohumeral joint is the most frequently dislocated joint owing to its poor stability (the glenoid cavity is small in relation to the humeral head); injuries usually result from a fall on the arm in forced abduction and external rotation, but can also result from a direct fall on the posterolateral shoulder. The humeral head and glenoid cavity may fracture (Hill–Sachs and bony Bankart lesions, respectively), and injury to the brachial plexus may lead to an **axillary nerve palsy** (leading to **inability to abduct** the arm due to deltoid paralysis and **hypesthesia** on the lateral shoulder skin). Associated **rotator cuff tears** also occur on occasion. In a posterior dislocation the anterior shoulder looks flat, the coracoid process is prominent, and the patient cannot externally rotate the arm.

Epidemiology

Greater than 85% of all shoulder dislocations are anterior (the humeral head lies in front of the coracoid process of the scapula); capsular tears predispose patients to recurrent dislocations. Posterior dislocations are less common and are associated with seizures and electric shock. Inferior dislocations are rare and occur when the shoulder is forcefully hyperabducted; when the arm is stuck pointing straight up this is known as **luxatio erecta.**

Management

Rule out fractures via AP, lateral, and axillary x-ray views before attempting reduction. Success of closed reduction is inversely proportional to time elapsed since injury. Analgesics are often sufficient for pain control, but sedation or general anesthesia may be needed for reduction. There are multiple maneuvers used to achieve reduction; the most common is the **Kocher method,** which involves applying traction on the humerus with the elbow at 90 degrees, **externally rotating** the arm, maintaining traction, and then **adducting** the arm and **internally rotating** it until a click is heard. **X-ray confirmation (including axillary view) is required to confirm reduction.** In young patients, **immobilize** for 3 weeks; in the elderly, begin range-of-motion exercises earlier to prevent stiff shoulder. **Recurrent dislocations** require soft-tissue/capsular surgical repair.

Complications

Recurrent dislocation, rotator cuff tear, lateral tear, humerus or glenoid fracture, axillary nerve injury, and brachial plexus dysfunction.

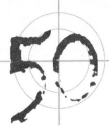

case 50

ID/CC	A 68-year-old man presents with **inability to fully extend** the fifth fingers bilaterally.
HPI	The patient is diabetic and has a history of **alcoholism** and **hepatic cirrhosis.** His symptoms are not painful and have been present and gradually worsening for years. His sister had similar symptoms that required surgery.
PE	VS: normal. PE: localized thickening of palmar fascia bilaterally with palpable longitudinal cordlike bands of tissue on volar aspects of fifth fingers extending into the palm and drawing both digits into flexion contractures; bilateral hands are otherwise fully neurovascularly intact.
Labs	CBC/Lytes: normal. Low albumin. LFTs: elevated AST and GGT.
Imaging	XR: no bony abnormalities; MCP and interphalangeal joints normal.

case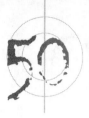

Dupuytren Contracture

Pathogenesis

The etiology of Dupuytren contracture is unknown; it is a disease of the volar hand fascia; there appears to be a **genetic susceptibility** in some families. The condition is **often bilateral,** and in severe cases may also involve the palmar fascia of the feet (LEDERHOSEN DISEASE) and the Buck fascia of the penis (PEYRONIE DISEASE).

Epidemiology

More common in older men; seen with increased frequency in patients with **cirrhosis,** in epileptic patients on hydantoin, in diabetics, and in patients status post-MI. It most commonly affects the fourth and fifth fingers. There is an early-onset form that occurs in patients less than 30 years old and seems to be associated with more severe symptoms.

Management

Early cases may be treated with **physical therapy,** night splinting, and gentle stretching. Injection of corticosteroid into the contracture may lead to dissolution. Advanced cases require excision or division of affected fascia. **Surgery** yields good results except when permanent joint changes have occurred in the MCP and PIP joints.

Complications

High rate of recurrence after operative treatment (15% to 20% recurrence).

Breakout Point

- Ring and small finger most commonly affected
- Thickening and fibrosis of palmar fascia
- Associated with antiseizure medications, cirrhosis, diabetes
- Lederhosen disease = thickening of foot plantar fascia
- Peyronie disease = thickening of penile fascia

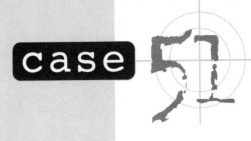

case 51

ID/CC	An 85-year-old woman was found down at home by her husband. She tripped on a rug, and is unable to **bear weight** on her left leg.
HPI	She tripped the previous night while walking to the bathroom in the dark, landing on her left hip. She complains of left groin pain exacerbated by any movement of the left lower extremity. Onset of **menopause** was 35 years ago. She is not receiving hormone replacement therapy or calcium supplements.
PE	PE: afebrile. Stable vital signs. Left leg **externally rotated, shortened, and adducted; positive logroll test, tenderness in left groin;** attempted hip range-of-motion testing causes her severe pain.
Labs	CBC: normal.
Imaging	See Figure 51-1.

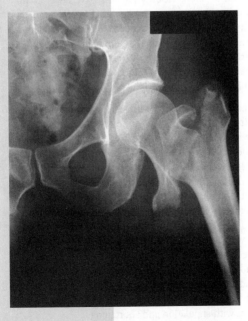

Figure 51-1. Anteroposterior radiograph of irreducible intertrochanteric fracture of the femur, necessitating formal open reduction.

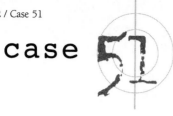

case

Hip Fracture

Pathogenesis

Osteoporosis is an important contributory factor to hip fracture in the elderly, in whom the fracture can result after a seemingly trivial fall. In young adults, hip fractures are usually the result of a high-energy injury such as a fall off a roof. Hip fractures are classified as **intracapsular** (subcapital [below the head] and transcervical [through the neck]) and **extracapsular** (basicervical [base of the neck] and intertrochanteric [between the greater and lesser trochanters]); the surgical treatment is different for each type.

Epidemiology

Most commonly seen in **osteoporotic elderly women;** however, elderly men are also at risk. Although they can occur in the young, 97% of hip fractures occur in patients over 50 years of age. Factors that confer a poorer prognosis are advanced age, poorly treated co-morbidities, male gender, and low level of function prior to fracture.

Management

The vast majority of hip fractures are treated operatively. Type of fixation depends on the specific fracture pattern and location. Healthy patients have fewer complications if they have surgery within the first 48 hours after injury. In rare cases, nondisplaced, stable, impacted femoral neck fractures can be treated nonoperatively in patients with serious co-morbidities that preclude surgery. **All hip fracture patients should receive perioperative anticoagulation for DVT prophylaxis.**

Complications

Hip fractures are associated with significant **morbidity and mortality**. The rate of **death** in the first year following hip fracture is in the range of 14% to 36%. The main blood supply of the head of the femur in the adult comes from retinacular vessels within the joint capsule, and these can be significantly damaged in intracapsular femoral neck fractures, leading to **avascular necrosis (AVN) of the femoral head.** Approximately 80% of displaced intracapsular hip fractures would progress to AVN and are therefore most commonly treated with a femoral head prosthesis (hemiarthroplasty). In general, extracapsular fractures do not damage the femoral head blood supply, and therefore have a low risk of AVN and can be treated using screws or rods into the native femoral head. Other complications include nonunion or malunion with angulation and shortening.

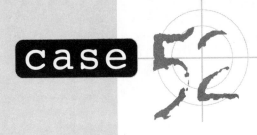

case 52

ID/CC	A **19-year-old male** college student complains of **pain** in the right knee and mild **swelling** of the thigh.
HPI	Otherwise healthy, he has been having **dull, aching pain** for several weeks that **worsens at night**. The pain is not relieved with aspirin. He denies any malaise, fever, chills, diaphoresis, headache, nausea, vomiting, or weight loss. Of note, he had a right eye enucleation at age 1 for retinoblastoma.
PE	VS: normal. PE: no acute distress; no jaundice; upper right thigh with **nontender** fullness, no **limitations of range of motion** at the hip or knee; no inguinal lymphadenopathy.
Labs	Elevated **alkaline phosphatase**. LFTs: normal. Immunoelectrophoresis normal (rules out multiple myeloma); calcium, phosphorus, and PTH normal.
Imaging	See Figures 52-1 to 52-3.

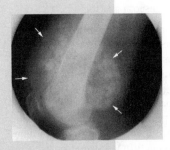

Figure 52-1.
XR, knee (lateral). **Osteolytic metaphyseal** lesion in the distal end of the femur cortical involvement with "sunburst" appearance (*arrows*).

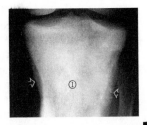

Figure 52-2. XR, knee (PA). A different case with speculated periosteal reaction and **dense sclerosis** (*1*).

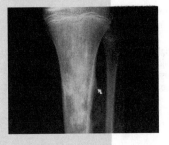

Figure 52-3. XR, tibia. Another case with lifted **periosteal new bone** in a triangular shape (CODMAN TRIANGLE) (*arrow*).

case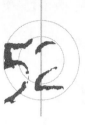

Osteosarcoma

Pathogenesis

Osteosarcoma, also called **osteogenic sarcoma**, is a primary malignant tumor of bone. Patients with **retinoblastoma gene mutations** who have undergone **radiation** are at highest risk for osteosarcoma. It affects **long bones** in the following order of frequency: **distal femur, proximal tibia**, proximal humerus, and pelvis. The prognosis is better for tumors in the tibia than for those in the femur. Patients may present with a **painless mass** or with **dull, aching pain following a minor injury.** Pain that is **worse at night** in a child is almost pathomneumonic for tumor. Pathology at the hip or proximal femur is often **perceived as knee pain**, especially in children. Articular cartilage provides a barrier to tumor spread. The tumor metastasizes most frequently to the lungs.

Epidemiology

The second **most common primary malignant tumor of the bone** after myeloma; usually affects **younger individuals** (teens) and shows no gender predominance. **Paget disease of bone** is a predisposing factor, accounting for the second peak of incidence in middle age. **Chronic osteomyelitis** is also a predisposing factor.

Management

Osteosarcoma can be lethal if not diagnosed and treated early with **aggressive resection** (wide surgical resection with reconstruction versus amputation) with **radiation therapy** and **chemotherapy.** Five-year survival rates with appropriate therapy range from 65% to 70%, but if the tumor is metastatic at diagnosis only 40% remain free of progression at 2 years. A possible primary tumor with bone metastases should be sought. Radiotherapy is much more successful in **Ewing sarcoma** than in osteosarcoma.

Complications

Pathologic fracture and **secondary infection; metastatic disease** (lung metastases) and **lymphatic involvement.** Death from advanced or metastatic disease.

Breakout Point

- Chief complaint of **night pain** is classic for tumor.
- Associated with retinoblastoma gene mutations in young patients and Paget disease in older patients.
- Bimodal distribution of peak incidence.

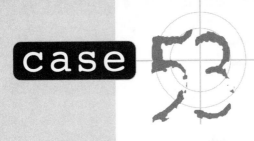

case 53

ID/CC A **10-year-old boy** presents with **pain in the right ankle and inability to bear weight on that side. He also has malaise, and fever** of 3 days' duration.

HPI Two weeks ago, he fell and **injured** his right distal shin; he initially had an open wound over the anterior tibia but this has since resolved. His mother reports that the leg has been swollen and warm. There is no family history of sickle-cell disease.

PE VS: **fever** (38.5°C). PE: **erythema, swelling,** and **tenderness** over right lower tibia; no open wounds, movement at ankle limited by pain; no crepitus or fluctuance.

Labs CBC: **leukocytosis** (16,500) with predominant **neutrophilia.** ESR elevated (68 mm/hr). C-reactive protein (CRP) elevated (130.3 mg/L). Blood culture yields *Staphylococcus aureus;* bone aspiration reveals frank pus, Gram stain shows gram-positive cocci in clusters and abundant neutrophils. Aspiration of the ankle joint yields normal clear yellow, sterile synovial fluid only.

Imaging See Figures 53-1 to 53-3.

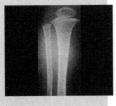

Figure 53-1. XR, right tibia. Normal initially.

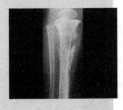

Figure 53-3. XR, right tibia. Periosteal **new-bone formation** at the upper tibial metaphysis.

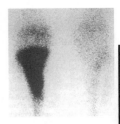

Figure 53-2. Nuc (technetium-99). **Increased uptake** at the proximal tibia in the metaphyseal area.

ORTHOPEDIC

case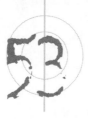

Osteomyelitis

Pathogenesis

Staphylococcus aureus is the most common organism responsible for osteomyelitis. The most common gram-negative organism is *Pseudomonas aeruginosa*. In patients with sickle-cell disease, *Salmonella* osteomyelitis is common. The organisms reach the bone via the **hematogenous route**. Suppuration occurs, leading to **bone necrosis**; pus forms under the periosteum, strips it, and penetrates through, forming a sinus. Necrotic bone is called **sequestrum**; the new subperiosteal bone that forms around the dead bone, forming a shell, is called **involucrum**. The **lower femoral metaphysis** is the most common site involved.

Epidemiology

Acute osteomyelitis is usually a **disease of childhood** and is more common among **boys. Immune-compromised individuals and diabetic adults** are also susceptible. Plain radiographs may be normal in the acute setting and MRI is required for further evaluation.

Management

Penicillinase-resistant antibiotics (e.g., nafcillin) in combination with an **aminoglycoside** for at least **6 weeks**; resolution of fever and decreasing ESR/CRP are good indicators of the effectiveness of such therapy. **If pus has formed at the site of osteomyelitis, it must be surgically drained with debridement of all necrotic bone.**

Complications

Complications of acute osteomyelitis include chronic osteomyelitis, septic arthritis (in joints where the metaphysis is intra-articular such as the hip), pathologic fracture (bone may be weakened by infection or surgical intervention), and growth plate disturbances leading to limb-length inequality.

Breakout Point

- *S. aureus* most common causative organism.
- Think *Salmonella* in patients with sickle-cell disease.
- Think *Pseudomonas* in patients with history of IV drug use.
- Frank pus within bone always needs surgical debridement.
- Treat with 6 weeks of IV antibiotics.

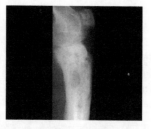

Figure 53-4. A different case showing chronic osteomyelitis with extensive sclerosis.

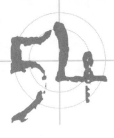

ID/CC   A 50-year-old woman presents with pain, swelling, and deformity of the left wrist.

HPI   One hour ago, she **fell on her outstretched left hand.**

PE   VS: normal. PE: tenderness and irregularity of lower end of radius with characteristic **"dinner fork" deformity;** radial styloid process palpated at level of ulnar styloid process (normally it is situated higher than the radial styloid); supination of distal fragment; no pain on passive extension of fingers (rule out compartment syndrome); palpable radial and ulnar pulses.

Labs   Not relevant.

Imaging   See Figures 54-1 to 54-3.

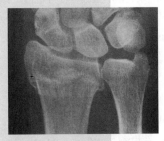

Figure 54-1. XR, wrist (PA). Disruption of bony trabeculae and cortical stepoff.

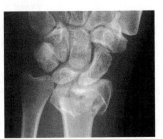

Figure 54-2. XR, wrist (PA). Intra-articular comminuted fracture.

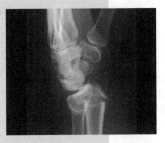

Figure 54-3. XR, wrist (lateral). The distal articular surface of the radius faces dorsally.

ORTHOPEDIC

case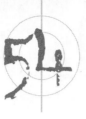

Radius Fracture

Pathogenesis	Distal radius fractures almost always result from **a fall on an outstretched hand.** If there is displacement, whether the distal fragment displaces **dorsally (Colles Fracture)** or **volarly (Smith Fracture)** depends on whether the palm was up or down at the time of the impact. As with any fracture, distal radius fractures can be displaced or nondisplaced, intra-articular or extra-articular, with or without comminution, and open or closed.
Epidemiology	Although distal radius fracture is the **most common fracture in individuals older than 40 years,** it is also very common in children and is frequently seen with rollerblading, trampoline, and bicycle injuries. In younger individuals the force required to cause the fracture is greater, and therefore there is usually a greater degree of associated soft-tissue damage.
Management	Treat via **closed reduction and splinting** followed by **casting** in 1 to 2 weeks when swelling resolves. Indications for operative treatment include intra-articular comminution, failure to obtain an adequate bony alignment with closed reduction, neurovascular entrapment, and soft-tissue interposition at the fracture site.
Complications	Complications include stiffness and edema of the hand, malunion with angulation, associated pain from subluxation of the distal radioulnar joint, median nerve compression symptoms, tendon rupture, and compartment syndrome.

Breakout Point

- Most common fracture in patients >40 years old.
- Mechanism: fall onto outstretched hand.
- Colles fracture = dorsal displacement of the distal fragment.
- Smith fracture = volar (palmar) displacement of the distal fragment.
- Intra-articular or unstable fractures need surgery.

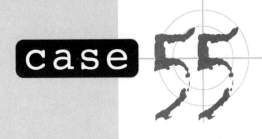

ID/CC A 40-year-old woman presents with an **acute onset of severe back pain.** The pain began while she was **moving boxes yesterday.**

HPI The pain worsens with movement, coughing, and straining (Valsalva), feels like a "hot poker," and **radiates to the right buttock and thigh.** She also complains of patchy **sensation loss** over the lateral right leg and a heaviness of the right foot causing it to catch on things while walking. The patient denies having any history of urinary or bowel incontinence.

PE Afebrile. VS normal. Low lumbar spinal tenderness with associated tenderness to palpation and paraspinous muscle spasm on the right; normal anal sphincter tone; no saddle anesthesia, no evidence of sciatica with straight leg raising; 2+ symmetric Achilles and patellar deep tendon reflexes with down-going toes bilaterally; decreased sensation over the lateral right leg and dorsum of the foot, three-fifths strength in resisted great toe dorsiflexion (L5 radiculopathy).

Labs Not relevant.

Imaging See Figure 55-1.

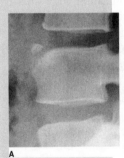 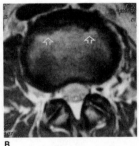 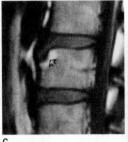

Figure 55-1. A. Lateral radiograph of the lumbar spine shows a typical appearance of limbus vertebrae. Axial **(B)** and sagittal **(C)** MR images demonstrate anterior intravertebral disk herniation (*open arrows*), but there is no evidence of posterior disk herniation.

case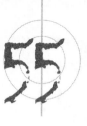

Lower Back Pain

Pathogenesis	This patient suffers from lower back pain due to degenerative disk disease. Degenerative changes of the annulus fibrosus and paraspinal ligaments may lead to herniation of the disk substance (nucleus pulposus) into the spinal canal; minor trauma is usually sufficient to precipitate symptoms. The herniation of disk material may compress one or more nerve roots, leading to **radicular pain** and to either **sensory or motor deficits.** The risk of nerve root compression is greater if the spinal canal is congenitally narrow or has become narrow as a result of hypertrophic changes in the facet joints. **Lumbar disk herniation most commonly affects the S1 nerve root** at the L5–S1 level **or the L5 nerve root (as in this example)** at the L4–L5 level, although extrusion of a large disk fragment may compress more than one root.
Epidemiology	Degenerative disk disease most commonly occurs in **smokers** and those exposed to **vibrational stress.** Also, patients who repeatedly **lift heavy objects** are at increased risk for back injury.
Management	Conservative treatment includes **complete bed rest, analgesia, traction, and mobilization in a corset.** **Surgical treatment** is indicated when there is bladder or bowel paralysis, muscle weakness, or failure of conservative therapy. Operative therapy includes surgical removal of the disk following laminectomy or chemonucleolysis (disk is dissolved with chymopapain).
Complications	Motor weakness, sensory loss, cauda equina syndrome, back spasms, persistent pain, and instability.
Breakout Point	

- Disc herniation pain worsens with coughing or straining.
- Symptoms of urinary retention, bowel incontinence, or saddle anesthesia are suggestive of cauda equina syndrome, which is a **surgical emergency.**
- Central disc herniations typically affect the spinal nerve root below their level; lateral disc herniations typically affect the nerve root at their level.

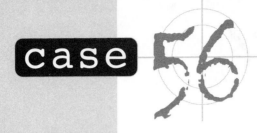

ID/CC	A 67-year-old male smoker with a 3-hour history of **sudden onset** of constant, **severe mid-epigastric abdominal pain** radiating to the back.
HPI	The patient denies gastrointestinal symptoms. He states he feels light-headed. The pain started while at rest. The patient has a **history of peripheral vascular disease** and is an insulin-dependent diabetic.
PE	VS: hypotension (90/60), tachycardia (120), afebrile. **Pulsatile abdominal mass** with **abdominal bruit.** No costovertebral or abdominal tenderness.
Labs	CBC with decreased hematocrit (32%).
Imaging	ECG: sinus tachycardia.

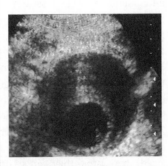

Figure 56-1. Abdominal ultrasound showing a large intraluminal clot within the abdominal aorta, free peritoneal fluid, and abdominal aorta 7 cm in **diameter.**

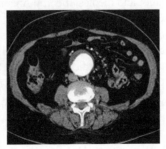

Figure 56-2. CT scan of the abdomen.

case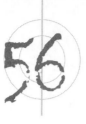

Abdominal Aortic Aneurysm

Pathogenesis

An aneurysm is defined as a focal dilatation with at least a 50% increase over normal arterial diameter. Abdominal aortic aneurysm (AAA) is a degenerative process of the aorta. The causes of AAA include **atherosclerosis (major risk factor)**, age, sex, smoking, hypertension, hyperlipidemia, peripheral vascular disease, myocardial infarction, family history, infection, arteritis, trauma, inherited connective-tissue disorders, and anastomotic disruption producing pseudo-aneurysms. AAA rupture likely occurs when the mechanical stress acting on the wall of the vessel exceeds the strength of the wall tissue.

Management

Two large-bore IVs with immediate **fluid resuscitation** and adequate oxygen saturation. Treat hemorrhagic shock with blood transfusion. Treat coagulopathy in patients on coumadin/heparin. **Immediate surgical treatment**—the aorta is reconstructed using either PTFE or Dacron. In patients who are diagnosed with unruptured AAA, elective surgical repair should be considered. Patients with symptomatic aneurysm should undergo repair, regardless of aneurysm size. Asymptomatic aneurysms greater than 5.5 cm in diameter should be repaired. For patients with medium-sized aneurysms, they can be managed with surveillance and medical therapy. Aneurysms 4.0 to 5.4 cm in diameter should be monitored by ultrasound or CT every 6 to 12 months. Aneurysms 3.0 to 4.0 cm in diameter should be monitored by ultrasound every 2 to 3 years. Medical therapy includes smoking cessation, beta-blocker therapy, and risk-factor reduction.

Complications

Death, MI, bowel obstruction, distal cholesterol embolization, and incisional hernias.

Breakout Point

- Ruptured AAAs have a very high mortality.
- In elderly male patients with renal colic, consider an AAA.
- Major risk factor is artherosclerosis

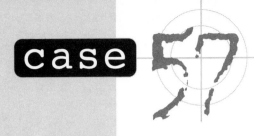

case 57

ID/CC	A 63-year-old man presents for a routine follow-up visit to his PCP and is found to have a **carotid bruit.**
HPI	He is an insulin-dependent diabetic and has a family history of **familial hypercholesterolemia.** He has a known 3.8-cm abdominal aortic aneurysm. The patient denies visual symptoms including a shade coming down over the eyes (amaurosis fugax) and other neurologic symptoms.
PE	Right carotid bruit.
Labs	Lipid profile: **elevated LDL.**
Imaging	Carotid duplex ultrasound showing a plaque within the right internal carotid artery. Contrast enhanced MR angiography confirmed the findings.
Gross Pathology	Not relevant.
Micro Pathology	Not relevant.

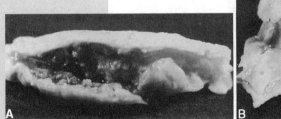

Figure 57-1. A carotid endarterectomy (CEA) specimen showing hemorrhage within an atherosclerotic plaque.

case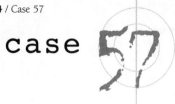

Carotid Stenosis

Pathogenesis

The proximal internal carotid artery and the carotid bifurcation are frequently affected by carotid atherosclerosis. Progression of atheromatous plaque can result in luminal narrowing and lead to **ischemic stroke** or **transient ischemic attack** (TIA). Other causes of carotid stenosis include aneurysms, fibromuscular dysplasia, arteritis, and vasospasm. *Amaurosis fugax* refers to transient loss of vision in one or both eyes. In patients with carotid stenosis, it generally signifies transient retinal ischemia.

Management

Carotid stenosis can be accurately diagnosed with **carotid duplex ultrasound.** MR angiography and CT angiography can also be utilized to evaluate the carotid arteries. Medical management includes risk-factor intervention, including management of hypertension, smoking cessation, blood glucose control, and use of statin drugs. Low-dose aspirin may be beneficial for patients who are high risk for stroke. Surgical options include endovascular and open techniques. Carotid angioplasty and stenting are best used for patients with high-grade stenosis. A **carotid endarterectomy** (CEA) should be considered in symptomatic patients with >70% carotid artery stenosis. Management of asymptomatic patients is controversial. CEA should be considered for medically stable men aged 40 to 75 years with asymptomatic carotid stenosis of 60% to 99%, and a life expectancy of at least 5 years, provided the perioperative risk of stroke and death is less than 3%.

Complications

CEA complications include stroke, damage to nerves (facial, vagus, hypoglossal, and glossopharyngeal), pseudoaneurysms, and MI.

Breakout Point

> In 100% carotid artery stenosis, surgery is not an option.

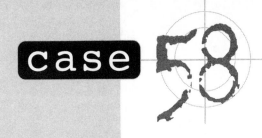

ID/CC	A 71-year-old male **smoker** presents with pain in both lower extremities on walking.
HPI	The pain occurs in both calves after walking 100 yards (claudication distance) and is **resolved with rest.** He has a history of insulin-dependent diabetes and hyperlipidemia.
PE	**Diminished peripheral pulses** bilaterally with a left femoral artery bruit. **Positive Buerger test**—foot pallor with elevation of the leg and a red flush spreading from the toes in the dependent position. Other physical findings include a cool extremity, increased capillary refill time, shiny colored skin, hair loss, and nail changes.
Labs	Increased levels of triglycerides and cholesterol.
Imaging	Ankle-brachial index (ABI) is 0.4.
Gross Pathology	Not relevant.
Micro Pathology	Not relevant.

case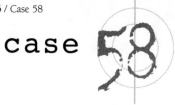

Peripheral Vascular Disease

Pathogenesis

Intermittent claudication is defined as reproducible lower-extremity discomfort that is induced by exercise and relieved with rest. It occurs due to an imbalance between supply and demand of blood flow to lower-extremity muscle groups. The majority of patients with peripheral vascular (arterial) disease (PVD) suffer from **peripheral atherosclerosis**; other causes of PVD include limb trauma, radiation exposure, and a vasculitis. Risk factors include diabetes mellitus, hyperlipidemia, smoking, and hypertension. Patients with **aortoiliac occlusive disease (Leriche syndrome)** may complain of buttock, hip, and thigh claudication, and impotence in men. Noninvasive testing, including **ankle-brachial index** (ABI) and segmental limb pressures, is used to diagnose PVD. Normal ABI is 1.0; ABI of 0.4 to 0.9 suggests peripheral vascular disease; below 0.4 suggests critical limb ischemia. Segmental limb pressures showing >20 mm Hg reduction in pressure between levels is considered significant. A lower-extremity angiogram can be performed for detailed arterial mapping.

Management

Therapy for intermittent claudication may involve medical, percutaneous, and/or surgical approaches. Medical management includes risk-factor management (smoking cessation, exercise, lipid-lowering agents). Surgical options include percutaneous transluminal angioplasty (PTA) or bypass surgery. If PTA fails or is not suitable, bypass surgery is performed.

Complications

Increased incidence of foot ulcers and poor wound-healing. Long-standing PVD may necessitate lower-extremity amputations.

Breakout Point

Site of Pain and Site of Arterial Disease
• Buttock and hip—aortoiliac disease
• Thigh—common femoral artery or aortoiliac
• Upper two-thirds of the calf—superficial femoral artery
• Lower one-third of the calf—popliteal artery
• Foot claudication—tibial or peroneal artery

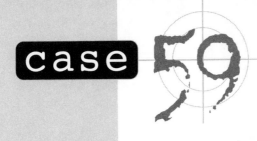

case 59

ID/CC	A 70-year-old man presents with worsening **right shoulder pain**.
HPI	He states that he noticed the shoulder pain 3 months ago and it has been getting worse. He also noticed right-sided **facial flushing** and **sweating** over the last few weeks. He has had progressive **fatigue, weight loss,** and **loss of appetite** as well. He admits to an 80 pack-year smoking history.
PE	VS: afebrile; tachypnea (RR 21). PE: no acute distress; barrel-shaped chest (underlying emphysema), **diminished breath sounds** in upper right lung field. Shoulder exam was normal. Mild right eye **ptosis, miosis,** and **enophthalmos.**
Labs	CBC: mild anemia (Hb 10.5 g/dL. Lytes/LFTs: normal.
Pathology	CT-guided biopsy showed non–small-cell lung cancer.
Imaging	CXR: asymmetrical opacity in the right lung apex.

THORACIC

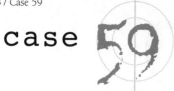

case

Lung Cancer

Pathogenesis

Lung cancer can arise as a result of a variety of caustic environmental agents, most notably **cigarette smoking**. Other causes include radon gas, arsenic, ionizing radiation, and asbestos (mesothelioma). Lung cancers are classified into small cell lung cancers (SCLC) and non–small cell lung cancers (NSCLC) based on treatment approaches. NSCLC include adenocarcinoma, squamous cell carcinoma, and large cell carcinoma and accounts for approximately 75% of all lung cancers. SCLC is almost always caused by smoking.

Epidemiology

Although lung cancer is **the second most common cancer in both men** (after prostate cancer) **and women** (after breast cancer), it accounts for the **most cancer deaths in both genders.** Lung cancer recently surpassed heart disease as the leading cause of smoking-related mortality.

Management

SCLC is classified into **limited-stage** or **extensive-stage** disease based on whether all of the disease can fit into **one radiotherapy portal.** Due to its propensity to metastasize, SCLC is treated with multiagent chemotherapy and thoracic radiotherapy rather than surgery. The staging workup for NSCLC generally includes CT of the chest, **mediastinoscopy to** evaluate the lymph nodes, and brain imaging to rule out metastases. PET/CT has shown to be helpful. Surgical resection is the primary and curative treatment for NSCLC. Surgical treatments include pneumonectomy, lobectomy, limited resection, and video-assisted thoracoscopic surgery (VATS). Adjuvant chemotherapy and radiotherapy have shown to prolong survival in high-risk disease. Unresectable disease can be treated with chemotherapy and radiotherapy.

Complications

Advanced disease can lead to **superior vena cava syndrome** (neck, arm, and face swelling and arm pain due to compression of the superior vena cava), **hoarseness** (due to recurrent laryngeal nerve paralysis), and **Pancoast syndrome** (apical invasion of the cervical sympathetic plexus and arterial and venous trunks, causing muscle wasting, arm pain, reduced pulse, engorgement of the jugular vein, and Horner syndrome [ptosis, miosis, anhidrosis, and enophthalmos] as in this case). Other complications include metastatic disease, paraneoplastic syndromes (e.g., SIADH), and airway obstruction.

Breakout Point

Leading cause of cancer deaths in both genders.

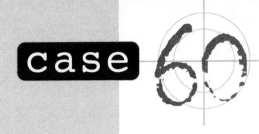

case 60

ID/CC An 80-year-old man presents to the Emergency Room with acute onset of severe **"tearing" chest pain.**

HPI The pain **radiates to his back.** He also reports onset of **voice hoarseness** just after his pain started. He has a history of noncompliance with his anti-hypertensive medications.

PE VS: afebrile, tachycardic (HR 110), **hypertensive** (BP 200/105), blood oxygen saturation 99% on room air. Heart regular rhythm with soft systolic murmur. Lungs clear. Chest wall nontender. Abdomen soft, no palpable masses. 2+ distal pulses throughout.

Labs Chemistries & CBC: normal. Cardiac enzymes normal.

Imaging Chest CT indicates clotted blood within the false lumen. ECG: normal.

THORACIC

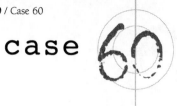

case

Aortic Dissection

Pathogenesis

Aortic dissection occurs when a false lumen is formed between layers of the aortic wall (intima and media). Propagation can occur proximal or distal. Thrombus can form within a false lumen, and there can be multiple communications between the true and false lumens. Traumatic dissection can also occur; classically this is the result of deceleration injury in a seatbelted motor vehicle accident victim. Aortic dissections are classified based on whether or not they involve the ascending aorta. The DeBakey and Daily classification systems are most commonly used. Daily **type A** involves the ascending aorta, whereas **type B** involves the descending aorta. The diagnostic studies of choice are chest CT angiogram or angiography. Dilatation of the aorta secondary to the false lumen filling with blood can cause stretch or compression of nearby structures and can lead to mediastinal widening on chest x-ray as well as voice hoarseness due to recurrent laryngeal nerve compression and Horner syndrome.

Epidemiology

Most common in patients 60 to 80 years of age with history of poorly controlled hypertension. Dissection can occur in isolation but frequently occurs in conjunction with secondary cardiovascular events such as myocardial infarction, stroke, or congestive heart failure. Aortic dissection is more common in people with collagen vascular disorders and with a history of cocaine use.

Management

Aortic dissection is a serious and potentially fatal condition. Patients need strict vital sign monitoring and observation. Daily type B dissections can be treated medically with blood pressure and heart rate control as long as the patient remains hemodynamically stable. Type A dissections generally require surgical intervention for repair of the intimal tear, stenting of occluded branching vessels, and aortic grafting.

Complications

Myocardial infaction, heart failure, aortic insufficiency, cardiac rupture, cardiac tamponade, death, splanchnic ischemia, limb ischemia, Horner syndrome, and recurrent laryngeal nerve injury.

Breakout Point

- Associated with uncontrolled HTN
- Type A = ascending aorta, surgical management
- Type B = descending aorta, medical management
- Pain classically "tearing," radiates to back
- Associated voice hoarseness and Horner syndrome

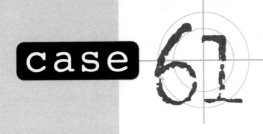

ID/CC   A 50-year-old **red-haired** man complains of a **bleeding mole** on his right arm.

HPI   The patient first saw the mole 2 years ago. Two months ago, he noticed the lesion had **changed color and increased in size.** The patient is a farmer (outdoor activity with **excessive sun exposure**).

PE   VS: normal. PE: **black-blue**, reticulated, **unevenly flecked**, hyperpigmented lesion on posterolateral aspect of the right arm; the lesion has an **irregular border**, a **raised, hyperkeratotic surface**, and faint erythema around the border as well as several small **satellite lesions**; numerous actinic keratoses on the patient's forehead and the back of his hands; right **axillary lymphadenopathy** noted.

Labs   CBC/Lytes/LFTs: normal.

Imaging   CXR: normal. CT: right axilla lymphadenopathy. Nuc: bone scan shows **metastases** to the humerus and pelvis.

SKIN

121

case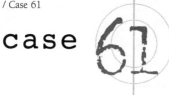

Melanoma

Pathogenesis

Malignant melanoma is associated with exposure to **sunlight** (UV radiation), with the greatest risk associated with acute, intermittent blistering sunburns, **genetic predisposition** (multiple lesions in families), and trauma (walking barefoot). The **ABCDEs** of melanoma are **asymmetry, border irregularity, color changes, diameter >6 cm, and elevation**. Warning signs include the recent appearance of a nevus or a change in a preexisting skin lesion, itching, pain, ulceration, crusting, bleeding, and rapid growth. The chief complaint in African-Americans may be zones of vitiligo (initially). Common sites include the **back** and lower leg (in women). There are four types. **Superficial spreading (most common), lentigo-maligna** (more common among the elderly), and **acral lentiginous** (affecting the palms, soles, and nail beds) all spread superficially and have a good prognosis. **Nodular melanoma**, however, exhibits rapid vertical growth (deeply invasive) and has a poor prognosis. In stage I and II disease (limited to skin), tumor thickness (Breslow depth) and presence of ulceration are the most important prognostic indicators. In stage III disease (nodal involvement), prognosis is influenced by clinical versus occult nodes, number of nodes involved, and presence of tumor ulceration.

Epidemiology

Melanoma constitutes **5% of skin cancers** and accounts for **two-thirds of all skin cancer deaths. Predisposing factors** include sun-sensitive skin type, immunosuppression, xeroderma pigmentosum, family history of melanoma, dysplastic mole syndrome, multiple common or atypical nevi. The overall 5-year survival rate is 80%; with positive lymph nodes it is 30%, and with distant metastases 10%.

Management

Excision is the treatment of choice for melanoma. Lymph node dissection is indicated in patients with clinical evidence of lymph node involvement in discrete drainage basins. Adjuvant therapy includes chemotherapy and radiation therapy, both of which result in partial responses in the range of 15% to 35%. Regimens using a combination of chemotherapy (cisplatin, vinblastine, and dacarbazine) and biotherapy (interferon-alpha and interleukin-2) have shown responses of up to 60% and increased survival in 10%.

Complications

Metastatic disease (e.g., to the brain); poor prognosis in disseminated disease.

Breakout Point

The ABCD Es of Melanoma	
Asymmetry	**D**iameter greater than 6 mm
Border irregularities	**E**nlargement
Color variegation (i.e., different colors within the same region)	

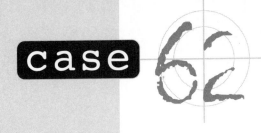

case 62

ID/CC	A 61-year-old man is brought to the ER with an extensively **painful, swollen,** and **erythematous** left lower extremity. Paramedics report that he is **febrile** and **tachycardic.**

HPI	The patient says that he sustained a small **laceration** on his left foot yesterday and that he noticed a small rash when he went to bed last night (**rapid progression**). He also has a history of **diabetes.**

PE	VS: temp 38.7°C, HR 139, BP 89/40, RR 24, O_2 sat 98% RA. General: **diaphoretic, pale, distressed;** musculoskeletal: **erythema** of left leg from knee to foot, turning a patchy **dark purple** color at the ankle, **blisters** on dorsal aspect of foot, **extreme pain** on palpation, crepitus felt under the skin of calf.

Labs	CBC: **leukocytosis with marked left shift.** Chem: **bicarb 17 (acidosis); elevated CPK 4300.** Blood cultures drawn.

Imaging	Conventional radiographs, CT and MRI can help to show **air** in the tissues as well as inflammatory changes; however **none of these studies should delay** prompt surgical exploration, which will clench the diagnosis.

Gross Pathology	Not relevant.

SKIN

case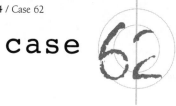

Necrotizing Fasciitis

Pathogenesis

Necrotizing fasciitis is a deep-tissue bacterial infection characterized by extensive tissue damage, rapid bacterial spread along fascial planes, systemic toxicity, and high mortality. **Type I: polymicrobial**, occurring after surgical procedures and in patients who are immune-compromised, diabetic, or with peripheral vascular disease. **Type II: monomicrobial** (often caused by group A Strep and, more recently, MRSA) can occur in anyone.

Management

Early and aggressive **surgical exploration and debridement** are the key to treatment for necrotizing fasciitis. Broad-spectrum **antibiotics** and aggressive **hydration** are also needed. **Re-exploration** is often required with the goal of removing all necrotic tissue. **Fournier gangrene** is a subset of necrotizing fasciitis occurring in the groin and perineal area, and may require cystostomy, colostomy, and orchiectomy for extensive disease. Hyperbaric oxygen and IVIG are still relatively experimental treatments of necrotizing fasciitis.

Complications

Systemic toxicity, shock, rapid progression, high morbidity, and mortality.

Breakout Point

Clinical Signs of Necrotizing Fasciitis

- Fever
- Intense localized pain
- Systemic toxicity
  Hypotension
  Tachycardia
- Crepitus

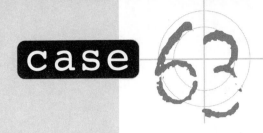

case 63

ID/CC	A 68-year-old man 24 hours postop noted to have **shortness of breath, total body edema,** and **ascites** coupled with low urine output and mild **hypotension.**
HPI	He underwent a partial liver resection (hepatectomy) for cancer. The duration of the surgery was 8 hours, during which he received 7,000 mL of IV fluid (lactated Ringer solution). The procedure estimated blood loss (EBL) was 1,000 mL and the patient did not receive supplemental blood transfusion for religious reasons. There were no signs of bleeding at the conclusion of the procedure.
PE	VS: afebrile, slightly tachycardic (HR 115), BP 98/60, pulse oxygen saturation 91% on room air. Body weight **5 kg above baseline,** JVP flat, diffuse **pitting edema,** skin cool and pale, diffuse rales throughout all lung fields, fluid wave on abdominal exam (ascites).
Labs	CBC: anemia (HCT 30%), albumin: 1.9. Chemistry: BUN 55, creatinine 1.9, bicarbonate 30.0 (mild metabolic alkalosis). Measurement of urine output shows 120 mL over the last 8 hours.
Imaging	CXR: diffuse perihilar infiltrate.

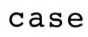 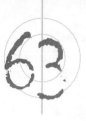

Fluid Status

Pathogenesis

This patient has simultaneous **total body fluid overload** with **third spacing** (peripheral and pulmonary edema) and **intravascular volume depletion** (tachycardia, hypotension, low urine output, cool skin). This can occur when intravascular fluid becomes depleted of high-osmolality components such as albumin. Normally, intravascular protein concentrations exceed interstitial concentration, so the osmotic pressure exerted by plasma proteins (colloid pressure or oncotic pressure) is higher than interstitial oncotic pressure and fluid remains within the vessels. If plasma oncotic pressure is decreased, fluid will tend to flow from the vessels to the interstitial space, causing intravascular volume depletion and extravascular edema.

Epidemiology

Most commonly occurs in critically ill patients in the hospital after surgery or trauma. Decreases in intravascular oncotic pressure can be caused by liver failure (low albumin production); or protein loss through surgical wounds or drains, ascites, or burns as well as dilution when large-volume crystalloid repletion occurs after surgery or trauma. In an ICU setting, volume status can be monitored very precisely with PA catheters, arterial lines, and central venous pressure monitors.

Management

Fluid management in this patient is complex. **The most important goal is to optimize end-organ tissue perfusion.** Vital sign trends are important in monitoring change in volume status after intervention. Other useful indicators of end-organ perfusion include peripheral skin turgor and warmth, mental status, urine output (normal U/O should be at least 0.5 mL/kg/hr in an adult), peripheral edema, laboratory studies, and imaging studies. Choice of IV fluid depends on the clinical scenario. In general, crystalloids (saline, Ringer lactate) are used for first-line resuscitation (rehydration) in the dehydrated patient. However, colloids such as albumin (5% or 25%) can be used to raise intravascular oncotic pressure and maintain intravascular volume while decreasing edema and third spacing. In the setting of clinically significant edema, colloid repletion is often coupled with diuresis to promote free water excretion by the kidneys. For calculations remember:

Total body water (TBW) = 60% × Total body weight (2:1 ratio intracellular volume [ICV] to extracellular volume [ECV])

Intravascular volume = 1/5 of the ECV

Complications

Dehydration, prerenal acute renal failure, respiratory distress secondary to pulmonary edema, wound and skin breakdown secondary to peripheral edema.

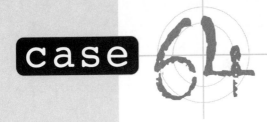

ID/CC A 28-year-old woman on **oral contraceptive pills** complains of sudden onset **shortness of breath** and **chest pain.**

HPI She is postoperative day two after open reduction and internal fixation of a **pelvic fracture.** While awaiting surgery, she was **immobilized** on bed-rest for 7 days. The pain in her chest is **sharp** and occurs on **deep inspiration** (PLEURITIC CHEST PAIN). She has also been coughing up small amounts of **blood-tinged sputum** (HEMOPTYSIS).

PE VS: low-grade fever (T: 100.8°F), **tachycardia** (HR 110), BP 116/82, **tachypnea** (RR 32), oxygen saturation 86% on room air, 92% on high-flow 100% oxygen. PE: moderate distress, lungs **clear to auscultation,** bilateral and symmetric breath sounds in all lung fields, no rales/rhonchi/wheezes, tachycardic but regular without murmur, chest wall and ribs nontender, no leg swelling, erythema, or cords (signs of DVT).

Labs CBC & chem: normal. D-dimer: five-fold elevation above normal.

Imaging Chest x-ray (not shown): clear lungs, no focal consolidations, pulmonary edema, or pneumothorax. ECG: sinus tachycardia, no other abnormalities.

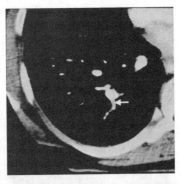

Figure 64-1. Spiral CT Chest w/ IV contrast, axial image, detail right lung. *Arrow* indicates small filling defect within subsegmental artery.

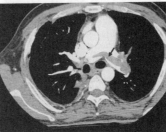

Figure 64-2. Spiral CT Chest w/ IV contrast, axial image. A different patient. Low-density mass (*arrow*) "Saddling" the left and right main pulmonary arteries.

OPERATIVE CARE/ANESTHESIA

127

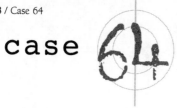

case 64

Postop Pulmonary Embolism

Pathogenesis

Pulmonary embolism (PE) occurs when **clotted venous blood particles embolize to the pulmonary vasculature and obstruct lung perfusion.** Most PEs originate from deep venous thromboses **(DVTs) in the pelvic and lower-extremity veins.** It is less common to have a thrombus travel from an upper extremity DVT to the lungs. Small PEs can be asymptomatic, whereas larger obstructions can result in respiratory distress, pulmonary infarction, pulmonary hypertension, right heart strain, and hemodynamic compromise, even death. The **Virchow triad of venous stasis, vessel wall injury, and hypercoagulability** describes factors shown to predispose to DVT formation. As hospitalized patients are at an increased risk, most are prescribed prophylactic doses of anticoagulant medications such as heparin for the time that they are in the hospital. Exposure to heparin can lead to antibody formation and result in **heparin-induced thrombocytopenia (HIT),** which is a procoagulable state and can increase risk for development of DVT and/or PE.

Epidemiology

The risk of venous thromboembolic disease (DVT/PE) increases with age, **immobilization** (bed-rest, neurologic impairment, air travel), surgery, trauma, **use of oral contraceptives or estrogen replacement, pregnancy, obesity, cardiac disease, and hypercoagulable state (malignancy, antiphospholipid antibodies, inherited).**

Management

Initial management of a patient with respiratory distress should include high-flow oxygen, chest x-ray, arterial blood gas (ABG), and ECG. The most common ECG findings with PE are nonspecific ST and T-wave changes, tachycardia, or T-wave inversions in the anterior leads (V1-V4). If chest x-ray and ECG do not reveal a cause of respiratory distress and/or there is an A-A gradient on ABG, then further studies should be done to rule out PE, such as **D-dimer or IV contrast spiral CT.** Once other diagnoses are ruled out, the treatment for PE is immediate systemic therapeutic anticoagulation with **IV heparin** or a similar agent. Severe PE cases can sometime benefit from the administration of intravenous thrombolytic therapy. Very large emboli (SADDLE EMBOLI) can be life threatening and may require resection of the clot (THROMBECTOMY) through surgery or percutaneous access of the pulmonary arterial tree. Anticoagulation with an oral agent such as Coumadin (WARFARIN) is typically continued for 3 to 6 months after PE or DVT.

Complications

Respiratory failure, intubation, right heart strain, pulmonary hypertension, death.

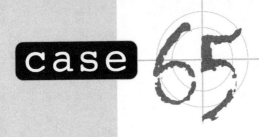

case 65

ID/CC	A 60-year-old diabetic man returns to the hospital, **5 days after** his **uncomplicated open cholecystectomy,** complaining of abdominal pain and fevers.
HPI	He was discharged home the day after the procedure. He did well until yesterday when he noticed **redness** around the incision site and a small amount of **purulent discharge. Pain** localizing to the same area began last night.
PE	VS: **temp 37.1°C, HR 80.** PE: cholecystectomy scar **intact,** with area of **erythema** and **induration** at the medial edge extending out 3 cm from the wound. Small amount of **pus** draining from the wound.
Labs	**WBC 16.4,** otherwise normal.
Imaging	Conventional radiographs are usually not useful in this instance. A CT scan can be used to evaluate extent of fluid collection within the wound and will often localize the areas of inflammation.

case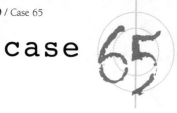

Wound Healing

Pathogenesis

Wounds are **weakest in the week following initial injury** and repair; after a month they may regain approximately 40% of their previous strength, 70% after 6 months, but may never be 100%. Despite sterile procedures and prophylaxis, surgical wound complications can occur in almost anyone. The most common complications are **hematoma, seroma, cellulitis, abscess, dehiscence, and nerve injury.** Antibiotics during surgery can help to reduce the incidence of infection. **Adequate tissue oxygenation is critical for wound healing and prevention of infection.** Neutrophils require significant levels of oxygen to produce superoxide radicals needed for bacterial killing. Tissue remodeling pathways such as collagen synthesis and many growth factor cascades are also highly dependent on adequate tissue oxygen tension. Suboptimal wound oxygen tension most commonly results from problems with **perfusion** (arthrosclerotic disease, smoking, hypovolemia) or **oxygen diffusion into tissues** (radiation-induced fibrosis, tissue edema, smoking). Other factors that negatively affect wound healing include **venous stasis, neuropathy, poorly controlled diabetes, poor nutritional status, direct wound pressure or mechanical stress on the wound,** and medications such as chemotherapeutics and steroids. A wound must be present for 3 months to be considered chronic.

Management

Treatment should start with a **thorough wound debridement** with removal of all necrotic tissue followed by **diligent wound care** until healing. Topical as well as systemic **antibiotics** may be indicated for associated bacterial infection. Hyperbaric oxygen treatment and **arterial revascularization** procedures can increase oxygenation to the wound. Strict elevation and compression dressings can decrease edema. Foot orthoses can be fitted to the patient to protect wounds on the feet from weight-bearing or pressure from regular shoes. Skin grafting or other surgical procedures are indicated only as long as the underlying processes that prevented healing have been identified and are appropriately treated; otherwise any new wounds or grafts will also be subject to poor healing conditions. The underlying causes of some chronic wounds cannot be corrected, and **amputation may be needed** as a last resort. These measures should be accompanied by tight glucose control. Smoking cessation and detrimental medications such as steroids and chemotherapeutics should be minimized until the wound is healed whenever possible.

Complications

Chronic infection, osteomyelitis requiring surgical debridement, abscess formation, systemic sepsis, and amputation.

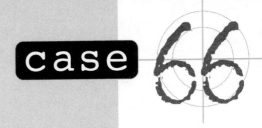

case 66

ID/CC	A 43-year-old woman has a fever of 100.5°F **one day** after surgery for ventral hernia repair.
HPI	She has denies chills, flushing, shortness of breath, burning with urination (DYSURIA), chest pain, or increased pain associated with her wound. She reports significant **abdominal pain** with deep inspiration and has subsequently only been taking **shallow breaths** since the surgery.
PE	Temp 100.5°F, HR 85, BP 115/85, oxygen saturation 98% on room air. Bilateral **basilar rales** on lung exam, no other focal findings. Abdomen soft, no rebound tenderness or guarding, appropriately tender around midline incisional wound. Wound clean and intact without erythema or drainage.
Labs	CBC: WBC 9.6, hematocrit 39.5%.
Imaging	Chest x-ray (not shown): no consolidation, effusion, or pulmonary edema.

case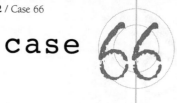

Postop Fever

Pathogenesis

This patient has postoperative fever likely due to atelectasis. The most likely cause of fever in a postop patient varies depending on the number of days since surgery. A **common pneumonic** for remembering causes of postop fever is the 5 Ws: **W**ind: atelectasis (POD#1), PNA; **W**ater: urinary tract infection (POD#3); **W**alking: deep vein thrombosis (POD#5); **W**ound: wound infection (POD#7); **W**eird drugs: medication-related fevers (secondary to antibiotics, neuroleptics, and a host of other medications). Delayed fevers that spike intermittently can be associated with abscesses. Blood transfusion is not uncommon after surgery, and transfusion reaction can also cause fever although this should be of short duration and resolve within hours of the transfusion being stopped.

Epidemiology

Low-grade postoperative fevers (<101.5°F) can be benign in many patients. Polytrauma patients, patients with long bone fractures, or patients following many orthopedic surgeries can have low-grade fevers for several days secondary to a heightened systemic inflammatory response to injury.

Management

Fevers in the first 48 postoperative hours are most likely benign and usually treated with Tylenol for symptomatic relief, deep breathing, cough, and chest physical therapy. After postoperative day 2, or in high-risk patients, fevers should receive a full workup. Standard initial fever workup includes physical exam, chest x-ray, blood cultures, sputum culture, CBC, urinalysis, and urine culture. Wound or drain fluid cultures can be included as appropriate. Failure to diagnose fever cause may require further imaging such as CT scan to rule out abscess and/or venous ultrasound to rule out DVT. In systemically ill patients with signs of sepsis, broad-spectrum antibiotics are often started while awaiting the results of cultures and imaging.

Complications

Occult abscess. Progression to systemic sepsis. Bacteremia with certain organisms (such as *Staphylococcus* spp. and *Streptococcus* spp.) can lead to endocarditis. Persistent high fevers can also increase insensible losses and lead to dehydration, especially in children.

Breakout Point

Remember 5 Ws
Wind: atelectasis (POD#1), PNA
Water: urinary tract infection (POD#3)
Walking: deep vein thrombosis (POD#5)
Wound: wound infection (POD#7)
Weird drugs: medication-related fevers

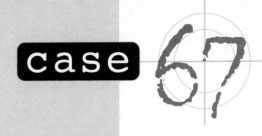

case 67

ID/CC A 46-year-old woman is found to have **muscle rigidity** and **skin cyanosis with mottling** 1 hour after a laparoscopic cholecystectomy.

HPI The patient received **halothane** anesthetic without complications. She tolerated her surgery well. In the postoperative recovery period 2 hours later, she had **masseter muscle stiffness**, increased CO_2 **production,** and skin cyanosis with mottling. She has no significant medical history and no known drug allergies. She is not on any medications.

PE HR 140, BP 105/65, RR 35, widened pulse pressure. Rectal temp 43°C.

Labs CBC: normal. Electrolytes: consistent with acute renal failure.

Imaging ECG: dysrhythmias, conduction disturbances, nonspecific ST-T wave changes.

case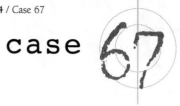

Malignant Hyperthermia

Pathogenesis

Malignant hyperthermia is a rare genetic disorder that occurs after administration of anesthetic agents, most commonly **succinylcholine** and **halothane**. The condition usually begins 1 hour after administration of the anesthetic agent but can be delayed up to 10 hours. Half of all cases are inherited as autosomal dominant and involve mutations in the gene for the skeletal muscle ryanodine receptor (RyR1), which leads to excessive calcium release from the sarcoplasmic reticulum in skeletal muscle when the offending agent is given. The body's metabolism suddenly increases, causing a sudden increase in core body temperature and muscle rigidity.

Management

Dantrolene is the main treatment and should be started as soon as malignant hyperthermia is suspected. It works by blocking calcium release. Supportive care, including fluid resuscitation and cooling measures. In-vitro contracture testing (treat muscle biopsy specimens in a tissue bath with either halothane or caffeine) for a definitive diagnosis.

Complications

Myoglobinuria, multiorgan system failure, complex dysrhythmias, rhabdomyolysis, electrolyte abnormalities, disseminated intravascular coagulation, acidosis, and death.

Breakout Point

- Succinylcholine and halothane are the common agents causing malignant hyperthermia.
- Dantrolene is the mainstay of treatment.

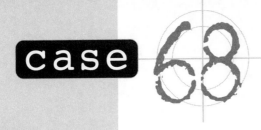

case 68

ID/CC A 42-year-old previously healthy woman presents with **severe headaches** with associated **nausea** and **vomiting.**

HPI The patients reports developing this new headache about 6 weeks ago. The headache is predominantly in the **morning** or when **lying down.** For the past 3 days, she has been waking up with increasingly severe headaches and vomiting.

PE T: 36.1°C, BP: 121/57, HR: 78, RR: 14, O_2sat, 98%. Cranial nerves examination shows impaired upward gaze. Fundoscopic evaluation reveals bilateral papilledema. Strength is full in all extremities. Sensation is intact. Reflexes are slightly brisk but overall and symmetric. Coordination is normal.

Labs CBC: normal. Chem 7: normal.

Imaging Pending.

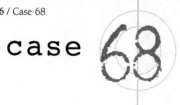

case

Intracranial Hypertension

Pathogenesis

Normal intracranial pressure is 15 mm Hg in adults, and intracranial hypertension (ICH) occurs when pressure is 20 mm Hg. Elevated intracranial pressure (ICP) occurs when there is increase in volume of one of the components: brain parenchyma, cerebrospinal fluid (CSF), or blood. Typical symptoms are **headaches and vomiting.** Other symptoms include **CN VI palsies, papilledema, spontaneous periorbital bruising, and the Cushing triad.** In this case, the pineal lesion is pressing on the tectum leading to obstruction of CSF flow, causing **Parinaud syndrome:** loss of upward gaze and convergence and possibly papillary dilation and loss of response to light and accommodation.

Management

The diagnosis of elevated ICP generally made on history, clinical findings, and imaging studies. ICP monitoring may be indicated in cases such as stroke, intracerebral hemorrhage, hydrocephalus, and subarachnoid hemorrhage. The best therapy for ICH is treating the cause of elevated ICP. This generally involves a surgical procedure, such as **decompressive cranioectomy, resection of tumor, CSF shunting, or evacuation of blood clots.** In urgent cases, always remember that the support of oxygenation, blood pressure, and end-organ perfusion is crucial to overall management. Medical therapies include mannitol, corticosteroids, hyperventilation, and barbiturates.

Complications

Herniation and death.

Breakout Point

Intracranial hypertension causes headache, vomiting, change in mental status, and papilledema.
Cushing triad for intracranial hypertension:

- Systemic hypertension
- Bradycardia with widening pulse
- Change in respiratory pattern

Emergent restoration of CSF flow or shunting is critical!

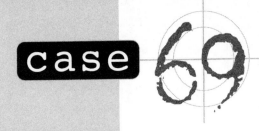

case 69

ID/CC   A 63-year-old man presents with **hoarseness**.

HPI   Patient reports 8-month history of painless **hoarseness** (dysphonia) that has progressively worsened. No dyspnea, dysphagia, odynophagia, or hemoptysis. He has a 50 pack-year history of **tobacco** use and continues to smoke cigarettes. He also has a history of heavy **alcohol** use. He denies symptoms of acid reflux or postnasal drip.

PE   Thin man in no acute distress. No cervical lymphadenopathy. **Fiber-optic laryngoscopy** reveals erythematous nodular lesions on the right vocal cord, which also has impaired mobility.

Labs   Thyroid function tests normal. The patient is taken to the operating room for a pan-endoscopy with biopsy.

Imaging   Chest x-ray is negative for lesions. Neck CT demonstrates laryngeal nodules on the right vocal cord and no significant cervical lymphadenopathy.

case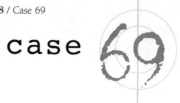

Head and Neck Cancer

Pathogenesis

Squamous cell carcinomas of the head and neck originate from the epithelial lining of the oral cavity, pharynx, and/or larynx. Risk factors include heavy **tobacco** or **alcohol** use, human **papillomavirus** infection, and a family history of squamous cell carcinomas of the head and neck. Field cancerization and multistep carcinogenesis are thought to play roles in the development of head and neck squamous cell carcinoma, as are mutations in **p53**.

Epidemiology

Squamous cell carcinomas are the most common type of head and neck cancers. They are predominantly found in **male** patients with at least a 2:1 ratio, and are also seen more commonly in patients **age >40**.

Management

Early-stage laryngeal carcinomas may be treated with **radiation** only, reserving surgical resection (partial or total **laryngectomy**) as an option for salvage if there is disease persistence or progression despite radiation. More advanced laryngeal carcinomas may require a more aggressive combination of surgery, radiation, and chemotherapy.

Complications

Untreated or inadequately treated laryngeal carcinoma can lead to **airway compromise** due to involvement and limitation of the narrowest point of the airway. Airway compromise can be managed with surgical resection, if possible, and/or tracheostomy tube placement. More broadly, it can also lead to local spread of the carcinoma above and below the vocal cords, as well as metastasis to cervical lymph nodes or beyond.

Breakout Point

- Persistent hoarseness or nonhealing oral ulcers should prompt a workup for head and neck cancer.
- Head and neck cancers are most common in men over age 40.
- Tobacco and alcohol use have a synergistic effect on the risk of developing head and neck cancer.

case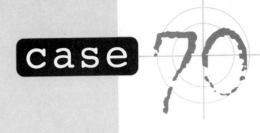

ID/CC	A 3-year-old boy with wheezing is brought to the ED by his mother.
HPI	The patient was running with some peanuts in his mouth this morning and fell. Immediately afterward he was noted to be coughing and choking, but he subsequently caught his breath. However his mother noted that he was wheezing and brought him to the emergency room.
PE	Well-developed, well-nourished young toddler in no acute distress. Coarse breath sounds bilaterally, decreased on right. Remainder of exam is normal.
Labs	WBC is mildly elevated.
Imaging	See Figure 70-1.

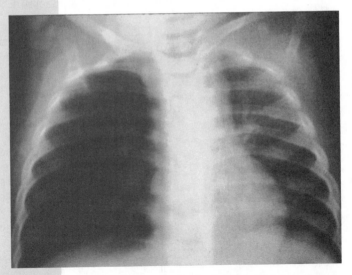

Figure 70-1. Chest x-ray shows **mediastinal shift** to the left and **hyper-inflation** on the right. No pneumothorax is visualized.

case

Foreign-Body Aspiration

Pathogenesis

This patient aspirated a peanut. **Foreign-body aspiration** can mechanically obstruct airways on expiration, resulting in air trapping as well as decreased air movement through a check-valve–type mechanism. With complete obstruction, consolidation can result after a period of time.

Epidemiology

Foreign body aspirations are most common in children over age 5, but can also be seen in adults. The tetrad of witnessed **choking, wheezing, unilaterally decreased breath sounds,** and **x-ray findings** has a 70% sensitivity.

Management

The definitive treatment is removal of the foreign body, usually through **bronchoscopy** in the operating room (Figure 70-2). Patients may also require antibiotics if they have developed a postobstructive pneumonia.

Complications

Complications can include inflammation, granulation tissue, and hemorrhage as well as pneumonia.

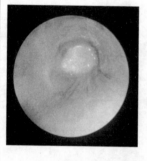

Figure 70-2. At bronchoscopy, inflammatory reaction to the obstructing foreign body in the airway was noted.

Breakout Point

Differential Diagnosis

- Asthma
- Upper respiratory infection with mucous plug
- Esophageal foreign body

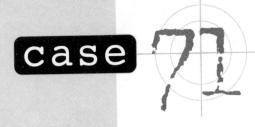

ID/CC A 48-year-old woman with a history of **inflammatory breast cancer** treated 3 years ago presents with severe **back pain** and bilateral lower-extremity **weakness** and **numbness**.

HPI She has been complaining of back pain for 4 months. Symptoms have worsened in past 5 days and she is nearly **incapable of walking**. She denies **saddle anesthesia, urinary retention,** or **fecal incontinence**.

PE T: 37.3°C, BP: 112/72, HR: 108, RR: 21, O$_2$sat: 93%. Midthoracic spine tenderness to palpation and percussion; upper extremities are full strength. Bilateral iliopsoas weakness 4-/5; otherwise, strength is almost full in lower extremities; reflexes are brisk; five-beat clonus and upgoing toes bilaterally; light touch sensation diminished in both legs, up to midabdominal level.

Labs WBC: 3.4, Hct: 30.2, PLT: 132.

Imaging See Figure 71-1.

NEUROLOGY

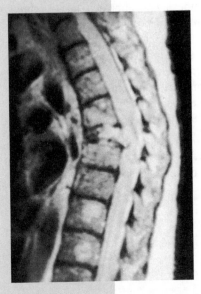

Figure 71-1. Epidural spinal metastases. T1-weighted sagittal MRI demonstrates destruction and collapse of the T6 vertebra. In addition to spinal cord compression from epidural extension of the neoplasm, there is a kyphotic deformity of the spine, indicating instability.

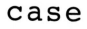 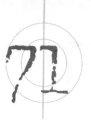

Spinal Cord Compression

Pathogenesis

Neoplastic epidural spinal cord compression is a **common complication of cancer metastases to the spine** that can cause irreversible loss of neurologic function. The three most common cancers causing spinal cord compressions are **prostate cancer, breast cancer, and lung cancer.** Renal cell carcinoma, non-Hodgkin lymphoma, and plasmacytoma or multiple myeloma are other significant causes. Spinal cord compression occurs when metastases or tumor invades the epidural space and compresses the thecal sac. Clinical symptoms include pain, motor findings, and sensory findings.

Management

MRI with contrast is the diagnostic imaging of choice in spinal cord compression. **High-dose steroids** should be given in suspected cases of spinal cord compression, even before diagnosis. In case of acute cord compression with otherwise good-performing scores, **surgical decompression** must be considered. Procedures include lateral approach for vertebrectomy and fusion and/or posterior laminectomy with possible fusion. The later is less invasive but risks destabilizing the spine further. Adjuvant radiotherapy is generally given to ensure local disease control. In patients with minimal symptoms, stable spine, and imaging diagnosis of spinal cord compression, radiotherapy can be the primary treatment modality.

Complications

Permanent loss of neurologic function.

Breakout Point

> Spinal cord compression is an emergency!

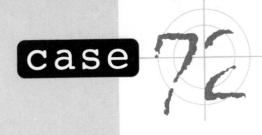

case 72

ID/CC	A 42-year-old man is brought to the emergency room after being assaulted and robbed. He sustained a **stab wound** to the abdomen during the struggle.
HPI	The patient has a history of hypertension, for which he takes metoprolol.
PE	**VS:** afebrile **HR 110, BP 78/52, RR 26,** O$_2$sat 98%. Chest: breath sounds equal bilaterally. Heart: **tachycardic,** regular rhythm with no murmurs, rubs, or gallops. Abdomen: **tender** in the right upper quadrant, **2-inch stab wound below the right coastal margin,** no external signs of bleeding. Extremities: **cool, clammy.** Neuro: alert, oriented × 3.
Labs	WBC nl, **Hb 9.3, Hct 32.4,** otherwise normal.
Imaging	Conventional radiographs show no fractures. **FAST ultrasound exam positive for free fluid** (likely blood) in the abdomen, with no pericardial fluid noted.

TRAUMA

case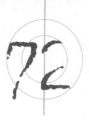

Hypovolemic Shock

Pathogenesis

Because of the body's compensatory mechanism, a fair amount of blood can be lost before classical signs of distress are evident, especially in a young, healthy individual. Loss of up to 25% of blood volume will cause mild to moderate tachycardia, tachypnea, and anxiety. Hypotension and confusion may not be present until over 30% of blood volume has been depleted.

Management

Patient must be stabilized immediately beginning with **airway** and **volume infusion**, as a search for the source of hemorrhage is initiated. Two **large-bore IVs** (16 gauge or larger) should be placed for access and infusion of **warmed crystalloids and blood** products. If IV access cannot be obtained, placement of a **large-bore central venous line** or venous cutdown should be initiated. A response in blood pressure and heart rate will signal the effectiveness and supports the presumed diagnosis, whereas lack of response may mean an active source of bleeding or another contributing factor. **Vasoconstricting medications** can be used as a bridging measure but the main goal of resuscitation is restoration of adequate volume and halting the source of hemorrhage. Clinical suspicion of an intra-abdominal bleed usually means immediate operative intervention (in this case, a liver laceration was found and repaired).

Complications

Inadequate volume repletion in the face of ongoing blood loss can quickly lead to **hypotension, loss of perfusion to vital organs (heart, kidneys, brain),** and **death.** **Lactic acidosis** can occur during large volume resuscitation and early airway intubation can help with respiratory compensation. Blankets and warming devices should be used to cover the patient to prevent **hypothermia.**

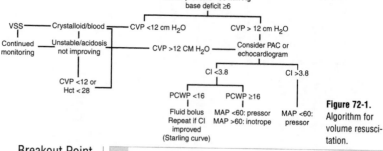

Figure 72-1. Algorithm for volume resuscitation.

Breakout Point

Goals of Resuscitation	
SBP > 90	CVP > 12 cm H_2O
MAP > 60 mm Hg	PCWP > 16
Hct > 28	

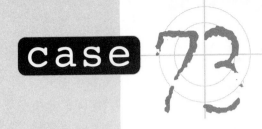

ID/CC   A 55-year-old man is bought to the Emergency Department after being rescued from a house **fire**.

HPI   He was found unconscious in his bed. His bed linens and pajamas were on fire. After 2 L of intravenous fluid resuscitation and supplemental oxygen he regains consciousness.

PE   VS: T 95.3°F, HR 101, BP 125/85, oxygen saturation 93% on 4L. Awake and talking. Singed nose hair and eyebrows. **Hypersensitive erythema** over face and neck. **Painful skin blistering** over left chest wall. Thick, leathery, asensate skin to right arm and right chest wall. Right forearm with circumferential burn. Right hand cool and pale, radial pulse weak. Left arm, back, perineum, and both legs spared.

Labs   Labs: carboxyhemoglobin 18% (normal 1–3%).

Imaging   **CXR: normal.**

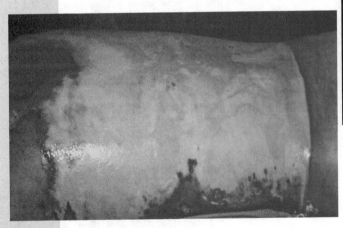

Figure 73-1. Full thickness burn.

TRAUMA

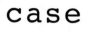 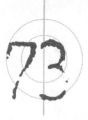

Burns

Pathogenesis

Burns are classified as full thickness (third degree) or partial thickness (second degree). First-degree burns involve the most superficial layers only (such as sunburns) and are not included in calculation of burn area. **Partial-thickness** burns tend to be **extremely painful** and are often characterized by blistering. **Full-thickness** burns involve all skin layers and result in pale, thick, leathery ASENSATE skin. The total area of skin affected by a burn can continue to increase for up to 72 hours after the initial injury.

Epidemiology

Increased age, TBSA of burn, proportion of full-thickness burn, degree of inhalation injury, and coexisting morbidities all result in higher mortality rate after burn injury.

Management

For minor burns the treatment can be as simple as the regular application of a burn cream such as Silvadene. Severe burns can require ICU-level care and months of reconstructive surgery. Initial care of a serious burn requires application of standard ACLS principles. A significant increase in fluid intake is required to counteract fluid losses through the areas of damaged skin. **The Parkland formula** (volume = 4 mL × TBSA × body weight [kg]) is used to estimate the total volume of fluid resuscitation a burn patient will require in the first 24 hours after injury. Large surface area burns can expose the body to significant ambient heat loss and patients often require hot rooms or heat lamps to avoid hypothermia. Circumferential burns of the extremities can require **surgical release (escarotomy)** to avoid occlusion of blood flow with swelling and subsequent limb ischemia. Most full-thickness burns (third degree) require surgical debridement followed by skin grafting. In the subacute setting, diligent wound care and infection control are extremely important. Chemical burns require copious irrigation or debridement to remove the toxic agent.

Complications

Limb ischemia, infection, sepsis, dehydration, skin graft failure, hypothermia, and death.

Breakout Point

> To estimate the total body surface area (TBSA) affected by a burn, the **RULE OF 9s:** the body is divided into 7 areas, each representing an estimated percentage of TBSA and each a multiple of 9: chest/abdomen (18% TBSA), back/buttocks (18% TBSA), arm (9% TBSA) × 2, leg (18% TBSA) × 2, and head (9% TBSA).

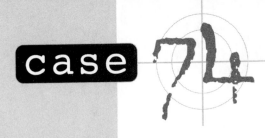

case 74

ID/CC	A 68-year-old woman who sustained mechanical **fall** complains of **headache** and **quadriparesis**.
HPI	The patient has a history of **rheumatoid arthritis.** She was found on the floor, complaining of **weakness in all extremities** and posterior headache. Her body and neck felt **numb**.
PE	Temp: 36.1°C; BP: 95/43; HR: 61; RR: 9; O_2sat: 91%. PE: patient's neck is in a hard collar. Cranial nerves are intact throughout. Strength in biceps and grasp is 3/5 bilaterally. She is otherwise **quadriplegic.** No sensation up to suboccipital area, which is very painful and above which sensation is preserved. Reflexes are very brisk, symmetric. Toes upgoing bilaterally.
Labs	WBC is 18.2.
Imaging	See Figure 74-1.

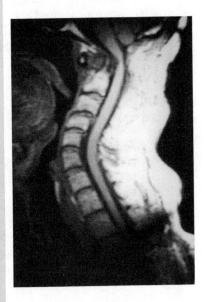

Figure 74-1. MRI of her cervical spine shows severe spinal stenosis in the upper cervical spine and cord compression.

TRAUMA

147

case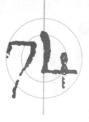

Cervical Spine Injury

Pathogenesis

This patient has an injury to the cervical spine. Most cervical spine fractures occur predominantly at **two levels: C2, and C6 or C7.** Most fatal injuries occur in upper cervical levels, either at craniocervical junction C1 or C2. C-spine injury can lead to mechanical instability, which may result in cord compression and neurologic damage.

Epidemiology

Cervical spine injury causes approximately 6,000 deaths and 5,000 new cases of quadriplegia each year. Approximately 5% to 10% of unconscious patients who suffered a motor vehicle accident or fall have a major injury to the cervical spine.

Management

Patients with suspected C-spine injury can be cleared with **NEXUS** criteria: no posterior midline cervical spine tenderness, no evidence of intoxication, normal level or alertness, no focal neurologic deficit, and no painful distracting injury. Otherwise, C-spine trauma series (x-ray) should be obtained. Patient's neck must remain in hard collar until cleared. In the case of confirmed C-spine injury, patient may require cervical fusion or other surgical interventions.

Complications

Spinal shock, neurogenic shock, autonomic dysfunction, permanent neurologic damage, and death.

Breakout Point

- Atlantoaxial subluxation can occur in up to 70% of patients with rheumatoid arthritis. About 11% will develop cord compression from the C1-C2 subluxation.
- High cervical cord compression will cause upper motor neuron signs and an ascending sensory loss with level. With severe compression, spontaneous breathing may cease and autonomic symptoms can appear.

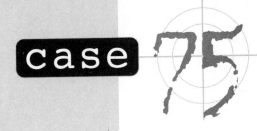

case 75

ID/CC A 25-year-old man was brought in by the ambulance due to **mental status change.**

HPI **Intoxicated** but otherwise previously healthy male was found unconscious in the street by EMT.

PE T: 36.1°C, BP: 146/85, HR: 105, RR: 18, O₂sat: 95%. Patient is somnolent, produces sounds only to stimulation. He does not open his eyes; his left pupil is 5 mm **nonreactive;** the right pupil is 3 mm, reactive to light. He does not follow command. In response to painful stimulation, he localizes with his left upper extremity, extends with the right upper extremity, and withdraws both lower extremities, the left brisker than the right one. There is a scalp laceration on the left parietal area.

Labs CBC: normal.

Imaging See Figure 75-1.

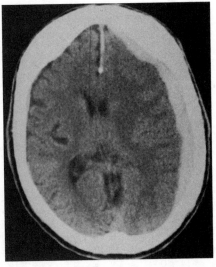

Figure 75-1. Noncontrast head CT shows a left hyperdense, crescent-shaped, extra-axial collection with mass effect (sulcal and ventricular effacement) and midline shift from left to right.

TRAUMA

149

case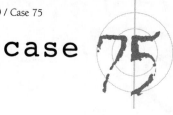

Head Trauma

Pathogenesis

Subdural hematomas often result from the stretching and tearing of **bridging veins** from the cortical surface to the venous sinuses. In traumatic cases, intracerebral contusions can also leak into the subdural space.

Management

An acute subdural hematoma with mental status change and neurologic deficit, significant mass effect on the brain and midline shift on CT scan, will need to be **evacuated emergently** by craniotomy. In this case, the left mydriasis is already indicative of uncal herniation and pressure on the left oculomotor nerve. A small, asymptomatic collection can sometimes be treated conservatively but will require observation, frequent neuro-checks, and serial imaging.

Complications

Herniation and death.

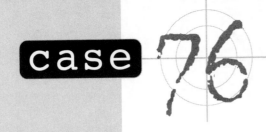

case 76

ID/CC   A 33-year-old man complains of **shortness of breath** and **chest pain** after a motor vehicle crash.

HPI   He was the unrestrained driver in a high-speed crash into a tree. Paramedics found him trapped between the seat and the steering wheel. His chest is covered in **multiple ecchymoses,** and there is an area that **moves inward** during inspiration **(flail chest).**

PE   VS: afebrile, HR 95, BP 136/78, oxygen saturation 94% on 4L. Awake and oriented. Chest wall tender with **bony crepitus,** area of **left chest that does not move** with the rest of the chest wall during inspiration/expiration **(paradoxical movement);** bilateral breath sounds present; lungs clear. Dark ecchymoses in the shape of steering wheel midchest. Heart regular rate and rhythm, no murmurs. Abdomen soft. No other injuries.

Labs   Chemistry: normal. CBC: normal. LFTs: normal.

Imaging   Chest x-ray (not shown): multiple fractures within each of the anterior left 5th to 8th ribs.

TRAUMA

case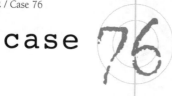

Chest Trauma

Pathogenesis

The major soft-tissue and organ injuries to consider in a patient who has suffered blunt or penetrating trauma to the chest are pneumothorax, hemothorax, lung contusion or laceration, cardiac contusion, cardiac tamponade, great vessel dissection or rupture, esophageal tear, bronchial tear, and diaphragmatic rupture. The bones of the sternum, ribs, and thoracic spine are frequently injured in chest trauma. Fractures of the sternum, first rib, and/or thoracic spine indicate a high-energy mechanism and are often associated with underlying organ injuries. **Flail chest occurs when multiple (at least three) adjacent ribs are each fractured in at least two locations,** resulting in a section of chest wall that is no longer in communication with the remainder of the rigid thorax. If the flail segment is large, it can severely compromise normal respiratory mechanics; patients may require intubation, and surgical stabilization is indicated in a rare number of severe cases. Even in the absence of a flail chest, multiple rib fractures are extremely painful and predispose patients to atelectasis and secondary pneumonia due to splinting and shallow breathing. **Pulmonary contusions** are very common after injury to the chest, and their magnitude is often not known until several days posttrauma. The clinical sequelae of pulmonary contusions can range from mild shortness of breath to pulmonary failure and acute respiratory distress syndrome (ARDS).

Epidemiology

Severe chest trauma is one of the leading causes of morbidity and mortality among trauma victims. Blunt chest trauma is most commonly a result of motor vehicle accidents. The top two causes of penetrating chest trauma in the United States are gunshot wounds and stab injuries.

Management

Initial management should follow **ACLS** principles (airway, breathing, circulation). Once the patient is stabilized, a portable chest x-ray should be performed. **A large hemothorax will be demonstrated by opacification of one hemithorax; pneumothorax can be detected by lack of lung markings.** Chest tubes should be placed for evidence of hemothorax and/or pneumothorax. The lung parenchyma often stops bleeding after re-expansion of the lung with chest tube placement. Surgical exploration of the chest is indicated if initial chest tube output is greater than 1,500 mL or if rate of continued output is greater than 300 mL/hr. Pulmonary contusions are frequently underestimated on initial chest x-ray and continue to evolve for at least 72 hours after injury. A chest x-ray with mediastinal widening, apical lung capping, and tracheal displacement is consistent with a mediastinal hematoma and should raise concern for traumatic great vessel rupture. All chest trauma patients should receive an ECG followed by an echocardiogram to rule out pericardial blood and heart injury if the ECG shows abnormalities concerning cardiac injury. Diaphragmatic rupture can be diagnosed by the presence of bowel loops or other abdominal contents above the diaphragm on chest x-ray. Diaphragmatic rupture requires surgical exploration and repair. Bony injuries to the clavicles, sternum, and ribs are generally treated conservatively with pain control and observation.

Complications

Respiratory distress, intubation, secondary pneumonia, atelectasis, and death.

questions

1. A 65-year-old man presents to the ER with moderate amounts of bright red blood per rectum, normal blood pressure, and normal heart rate. The first step in his management is:

   A. Check CBC
   B. Type and cross
   C. Insert two large bore IVs and begin fluid resuscitation
   D. Colonoscopy
   E. Insertion of nasogastric tube

2. A 45-year-old man suffered third-degree burns to 25% of his body surface due to a house fire. He develops fever and black patches in the burn wounds on ICU day 5. Which of the organisms is the most likely to cause his symptoms?

   A. *Staphylococcus aureus*
   B. Group A *Streptococcus*
   C. *Candida albicans*
   D. *Pseudomonas aeruginosa*
   E. Group B *Streptococcus*

3. A 65-year-old woman presents with "swelling" of the left breast. On exam, she has diffuse swelling around the left nipple, and the skin overlying the left breast is diffusely warm, erythematous, and indurated. This patient has:

   A. Mastitis
   B. Breast abscess
   C. Phyllodes tumor
   D. Paget's disease of the breast
   E. Inflammatory breast cancer

4. A 52-year-old man develops postprandial palpitations, sweating, diarrhea, and flushing of the face several months after a Billroth II procedure for peptic ulcer disease. The most likely cause is:

   A. Afferent loop syndrome
   B. Dumping syndrome
   C. Chronic pancreatitis
   D. Zollinger-Ellison syndrome
   E. Gastrointestinal hemorrhage

5. A 35-year-old man was sprinting and had to suddenly change direction due to traffic. He heard a pop in his left knee, and then experienced sudden onset of left knee pain and left knee fluctuant swelling. What's the most likely injury?

   A. Anterior cruciate ligament injury
   B. Lateral collateral ligament injury
   C. Medial collateral ligament injury
   D. Posterior cruciate ligament injury
   F. Prepatellar bursitis

6. A 60-year-old man with a history of diabetes returns to the clinic due to tongue pain. He was seen 2 months ago for similar complaint. The pain is worse now despite a course nystatin solution treatment. He continues to smoke two packs of cigarettes and drink 3 beers per day. On exam, his tongue ulcer seems to be smaller but deeper. What's the likely diagnosis?

   A. *Candida* infection
   B. Aphthous ulcers
   C. Behçet disease
   D. Herpes simplex infection
   E. Squamous cell cancer

7. A 50-year-old woman with a history of metastatic breast cancer presents to the ER with severe low back pain, and progressive weakness and numbness of bilateral lower extremities. In the ER, she tells you that she has not urinated for 18 hours. After foley catheter insertion, the patient put out 1,100 cc of urine. On exam, she has saddle anesthesia and bilateral lower extremity sensory deficit; 3/5 in both lower extremities. Rectal exam shows poor rectal tone. What is the most appropriate next step in management?

   A. Give high-dose steroids
   B. Obtain an MRI of the spine
   C. Consult neurosurgery for emergency decompression
   D. Consult radiation oncology for urgent radiotherapy
   E. Obtain a CT of the spine

8. A 70-year-old man with a history of diverticulosis presents to the ED with fever and abdominal pain. He had a sudden onset of pain and he describes the pain as diffuse. On exam, he is tachycardic and tachypneic, with a temperature of 38.5°C. Abdominal exam showed a rigid, board-like abdomen with generalized tenderness and hypoactive bowel sounds. Laboratory studies revealed a hemoglobin of 12.5 g/dl and a leukocyte count of 17,000/mm^3. What is the most likely diagnosis?

A. Diverticulitis

B. Acute small bowel obstruction

C. Acute large bowel obstruction

D. Perforated bowel

E. Severe gastroenteritis

9. A 60-year-old man comes to the office complaining of blood in the urine. He tells you that there is no pain associated with the blood and has occurred several times in the last month. Urinalysis showed 12–15 red blood cells, no white cells, and negative for nitrite and leukocyte esterase. Cystoscopy showed a 0.5-cm sessile lesion over the trigone. Pathology will most likely show:

A. Squamous cell carcinoma

B. Adenocarcinoma

C. Transitional cell carcinoma

D. Clear cell carcinoma

E. Chronic cystitis

10. A 32-year-old woman presents to the ED after an episode of hematemesis. She tells you that she went on an alcohol binge last night, which led to persistent vomiting. She saw some blood in the last episode of vomiting. The patient likely has:

A. Esophageal varices

B. Boerhaave syndrome

C. Peptic ulcer disease

D. Mallory-Weiss tear

E. Hepatic cirrhosis

11. A 50-year-old man undergoes a left hip replacement. Two days after admission, he develops anxiety, tremors, hallucinations, and had one episode of generalized seizure. What is the most likely diagnosis?

A. Pulmonary embolism

B. Delirium tremens

C. Postoperative psychosis

D. Hypoglycemia

E. Reaction to pain medications

12. A 20-year-old man fell while speeding his bicycle downhill. His abdomen hit the handlebar during the fall. He now complains of vague abdominal pain and some bruising of the anterior abdominal wall. His vital signs are stable and there are no other visible injuries. X-ray of the abdomen shows retroperitoneal air. What is the most likely diagnosis?

A. Abdominal contusion
B. Ruptured spleen
C. Hematoma in the abdominal muscle
D. Ruptured duodenum
E. Ruptured liver

13. A 25-year-old man sustained an injury to the lateral aspect of his right knee from a ski accident. He was unable to evert the foot effectively after the injury. What nerve did he injure?

    A. Anterior tibial nerve
    B. Posterior tibial nerve
    C. Sciatic nerve
    D. Peroneal nerve
    E. Obturator nerve

14. Which of the following is removed in a radical mastectomy, but not in a modified radical mastectomy?

    A. The nipple-areolar complex
    B. Axillary nodes
    C. Pectoralis minor
    D. Pectoralis major
    E. Supraclavicular lymph nodes

15. 43-year-old construction worker fell while walking along a steel beam, straddling the beam. He was brought to the ED with complaints of genital pain. On exam, he has a butterfly pattern of ecchymosis over the perineum. His bladder is palpable and he has gross blood at the urethral meatus. He wants to urinate but only a few drops of blood appear at the meatus when he tries. The next best step in management is:

    A. Insert a Foley catheter
    B. Obtain a scrotal ultrasound
    C. Obtain an abdominal/pelvic CT
    D. Obtain an abdominal/pelvic MRI
    E. Obtain a retrograde urethrogram

16. You see a 37-year-old, otherwise healthy, woman who complains of abdominal pain. On further questioning she reveals increased abdominal girth with a marked increase in her waist size over the last couple of months. On examination you note a full abdomen with a fluid wave, hepatomegaly, and tenderness in right upper quadrant. Labs reveal a normal liver panel, normal amylase and lipase, low WBC, and a low albumin. An ultrasound confirms ascites, and peritoneal fluid obtained via paracentesis reveals >3 g protein per deciliter. The most likely diagnosis is:

A. Alcoholic cirrhosis
B. Acute pancreatitis
C. Budd-Chiari syndrome
D. Congestive heart failure
E. Acute splenic rupture

17. A 12-year-old boy presents to clinic complaining of left thigh swelling and pain. He tells you that he remembers injuring his left thigh two months ago during a soccer game. He has a small contusion that went away after several days. However, he noticed left thigh pain and swelling 1 month ago. It has been gradually worse since. On exam, you noticed the boy's left thigh is much bigger than the right. X-ray shows a mass involving the left femur. The mass involves the femur and there is periosteal reaction, simulating "onion peel" appearance. What's the most likely diagnosis?

    A. Ewing sarcoma
    B. Osteosarcoma
    C. Hematoma
    D. Rhabdomyosarcoma
    E. Osteomyelitis

18. A 46-year old homeless man comes to the emergency department complaining of crampy, epigastric pain. This pain began about two weeks ago when he had a couple days of diarrhea (which resolved) and has been steadily worsening since that time. The pain is worst after eating and he feels full after only a couple of bites. On review of systems, he reports that a month ago he was involved in an altercation and was hit several times in the abdomen but did not come to the hospital afterward because he was feeling okay. He also reports some recent weight loss that he attributes to decreased appetite. On physical exam, he is afebrile and a deep, nontender mass is felt in the epigastric area. The patient is guaiac negative. What is the most likely cause of his problem?

    A. Abdominal aneurysm
    B. Gastritis
    C. Crohn disease
    D. Pancreatic pseudocyst
    E. Colitis

19. You are called to evaluate fever (101.3°F) in a 34-year-old man who is recovering in bed after surgery for appendicitis. Laparoscopic surgery was unsuccessful (unable to find appendix) and was converted to an open surgery, which was successful in removing his inflamed appendix. He has been unable to move around secondary to pain and you notice that there is no incentive spirometer at his bedside. Leaving the patient, you order incentive spirometry every hour as well as ambulation with assistance as soon as possible. The next evening, you are called again because the patient has spiked a fever to 101.5°F. The nurses report that he has been sleeping a lot because of pain medicine and has barely ambulated. Examination of his surgical wound reveals a clean, non-erythematous, non-tender wound that is healing well. What is the most likely next step in management for this patient?

A. Urinalysis, urine culture, and antibiotics
B. Ultrasound of the lower extremities to check for deep vein thrombosis
C. Chest x-ray, sputum cultures, and antibiotics
D. Abdominal CT scan
E. Reexploration in the OR

20. A 22-year-old chef is brought to the emergency room after tripping and falling onto a paring knife, sustaining a wound to his left upper chest. He sustained minimal blood loss before the paramedics arrived. He feels well upon being wheeled in and is speaking in full sentences. His pulse and blood pressure are stable, but he is breathing at a rate of 36. On physical examination, you find that there are no breath sounds on the left side, and the nurse tells you that his oxygen saturation is 88% on room air. What is the next step in the care of this trauma patient?

A. Chest x–ray
B. Chest CT
C. Rapid sequence intubation
D. IV fluids
E. Diagnostic peritoneal lavage

answers

1-C

   A. In an acute bleed, the CBC [Incorrect] may not show a decrease in hematocrit, since hematocrit is the concentration of red blood cells (total body blood volume decreases immediately due to hemorrhage, but concentration of red blood cells does not immediately change).

   B. Type and cross [Incorrect] is the next (second) step in management of GI bleeding, to prepare for possible red blood cell transfusion.

   C. The first step in the management of GI bleeding is insertion of two large-bore IVs and fluid resuscitation [Correct].

   D. Colonoscopy [Incorrect] would not be performed emergently in this patient, because his vital signs are normal.

   E. Insertion of nasogastric tube [Incorrect] is not performed as the first step in treatment, but is eventually done to determine whether the GI bleed is from the upper GI tract or the lower GI tract.

2-D

   A. *Staphylococcus aureus* [Incorrect] may infect burns, but is not the most commonly implicated organism.

   B. Group A *Streptococcus* [Incorrect] may infect burns, but is not the most commonly implicated organism.

   C. *Candida albicans* [Incorrect] may infect burns, but is not the most commonly implicated organism.

   D. Infection is the most common complication of burn injury. *Pseudomonas aeruginosa* [Correct] is the organism most frequently involved in burn infection.

   E. Group B *Streptococcus* [Incorrect] may infect burns, but is not the most commonly implicated organism.

3-E

   A. Mastitis [Incorrect] is a localized cellulitis (skin infection) precipitated by bacterial invasion through a fissured nipple; mastitis most commonly occurs in women who are breastfeeding.

   B. Breast abscess [Incorrect] is a potential complication of mastitis.

C. Phyllodes tumor [Incorrect] is a benign, usually very large (average size 5 cm), firm, mobile, well-circumscribed breast tumor; it is uncommon that Phyllodes tumor affects the overlying skin of the breast.

D. Paget disease of the breast [Incorrect] is defined by the finding of scaling, eczematous skin in the nipple/areolar complex. It is associated with underlying breast cancer.

E. Inflammatory breast cancer [Correct] is a clinical diagnosis in older women. It is defined as diffuse brawny induration of the skin of the breast with an erysipeloid edge, usually without an underlying palpable mass. The skin over the breast is warm, thickened, with a "peau d'orange" (skin of an orange) appearance.

4-B

A. Afferent loop syndrome [Incorrect] is a complication of Billroth II (gastrojejunostomy), characterized by postprandial fullness which is relieved by vomiting of bilious material. The afferent blind loop refers to the limb containing duodenum and proximal jejunum, which lies upstream from a gastrojejunostomy.

B. Dumping syndrome [Correct] is characterized by palpitations, sweating, diarrhea, and facial flushing shortly after meals. The etiology of dumping syndrome is not clear, but is likely associated with reactive hypoglycemia.

C. Chronic pancreatitis [Incorrect] can be associated with peptic ulcer disease, but epigastric pain is a more common presentation of pancreatitis.

D. Zollinger–Ellison syndrome [Incorrect] is characterized by the triad of severe peptic ulcer disease, non-beta pancreatic islet cell tumor, and gastric acid hypersecretion.

E. Gastrointestinal hemorrhage [Incorrect] is not the most likely cause of the above post-Billroth II symptoms.

5-A

A. Anterior cruciate ligament (ACL) injury [Correct] generally occurs when a runner suddenly changes direction, or when an athlete is hit from behind, such that his upper leg moves forward relative to the lower leg. Hearing a popping sound is pathognomonic of this condition. Hemarthrosis and immediate knee swelling are also common because the artery to the ACL runs along the ligament. Treatment is surgical repair.

B. Lateral collateral ligament injury [Incorrect] occurs when impact to the medial side of the knee induces the knee to be pushed out laterally (varus stress).

C. Medial collateral ligament injury [Incorrect] occurs when impact to the lateral side of the knee induces the knee to be pushed in medially (valgus stress).

D. The posterior collateral ligament [Incorrect] can be injured when an athlete falls on a bent knee, or if the bent knee is struck inferior to the patella on the dashboard during a motor vehicle accident (lower leg moves posterior relative to upper leg).

E. Prepatellar bursitis [Incorrect] occurs in plumbers, house-maids, and workers who spend a lot of time on their knees, such that the bursa on top of the patella becomes inflamed and painful.

6-E

A. *Candida* infection [Incorrect] should have been treated by nys-tatin solution.

B. Aphthous ulcers [Incorrect] do not last 2 months, though they can be recurrent.

C. Behçet disease is a chronic inflammatory condition character-ized by recurrent oral aphthae and systemic manifestations including genital aphthae, ocular disease, skin lesions, neuro-logic disease, vascular disease, or arthritis. In Behçet disease, oral ulcers tend to be multiple and extensive. Behçet disease is less common in smokers.

D. Herpes simplex infection [Incorrect] does not last 2 months, though it can be recurrent.

E. The patient's heavy smoking and alcohol history make him very high risk for squamous cell carcinoma [Correct] of the head and neck region.

7-A

A. The patient has symptoms of cauda equina syndrome, likely from breast cancer metastatic to the spine, causing thecal sac compression. The first step in management should be high-dose steroid therapy [Correct].

B. MRI of the spine [Incorrect] is the next step to determine the level and extent of disease (MRI shows more detail than CT).

C. In patients with progressive neurologic symptoms, emergency surgical decompression [Incorrect] is the treatment of choice.

D. Urgent radiotherapy [Incorrect] is another therapeutic option in spinal cord compression.

E. An MRI would show more detail than a CT of the spine [Incorrect].

8-D

 A. Given the patient's history of diverticulosis, perforated diverticulum [Incorrect] is the most likely cause of peritonitis.
 B. Small bowel obstruction [Incorrect] is most commonly caused by postsurgical adhesions, followed by Crohn disease, malignancy, and hernias.
 C. Large bowel obstruction causes abdominal distension and vague, crampy abdominal pain.
 D. The patient has signs of perforated bowel [Correct] and peritonitis, with an acute surgical board-like abdomen.
 E. Severe gastroenteritis [Incorrect] classically presents with diarrhea with or without vomiting and abdominal pain.

9-C

 A. Only 5% of all bladder tumors are squamous cell carcinoma [Incorrect].
 B. Only 2% of all bladder tumors are adenocarcinoma [Incorrect].
 C. More than 90% of all bladder tumors are transitional cell carcinoma [Correct].
 D. Clear cell carcinoma [Incorrect] is the most common malignancy of the kidney; histology shows small nuclei and abundant cytoplasm.
 E. Chronic cystitis [Incorrect] is associated with recurrent urinary tract infection and is treated with antibiotics.

10-D

 A. Esophageal varices [Incorrect] is an incorrect diagnosis in this case.
 B. Boerhaave syndrome [Incorrect] is spontaneous rupture of the esophagus associated with persistent retching and vomiting; the classic presentation is sudden, severe chest pain and subcutaneous emphysema (hematemesis is uncommon).
 C. There is no evidence to suggest this patient has peptic ulcer disease [Incorrect].
 D. A Mallory-Weiss tear [Correct] is characterized by an upper GI bleed due to mucosal lacerations at the gastroesophageal junction or gastric cardia. It is associated with persistent retching and vomiting.
 E. There is no evidence to suggest that this patient has cirrhosis [Incorrect].

11-B

A.

B. Symptoms of delirium tremens (DTs) include tremors, irritability, insomnia, nausea/vomiting, hallucinations, confusion, delusions, severe agitation, and seizures; DTs can result in death if untreated. Delirium tremens and alcohol withdrawal occur 48 hours after stopping alcohol intake. Many patients hide their alcohol history from their physicians. It is important to recognize signs of alcohol withdrawal as early as possible, because early intervention can prevent complications.

C.

12-D

A. Abdominal contusion [Incorrect] does not typically result in retroperitoneal air on abdominal imaging.

B. Ruptured spleen [Incorrect] does not typically result in retroperitoneal air on abdominal imaging.

C. Hematoma in the abdominal muscle [Incorrect] does not typically result in retroperitoneal air on abdominal imaging.

D. Patients with duodenal rupture [Correct] have vague symptoms because it is retroperitoneal. Retroperitoneal air on x-ray is the sine qua non of duodenal rupture. Motor vehicle accidents can cause duodenal rupture in children through lap belt injury; duodenal rupture in the driver can also occur as a result of compression against the steering wheel.

E. Ruptured liver [Incorrect] does not typically result in retroperitoneal air on abdominal imaging.

13-D

A. The anterior tibial nerve [Incorrect] does not cause the described symptoms.

B. The posterior tibial nerve [Incorrect] does not cause the described symptoms.

C. The sciatic nerve [Incorrect] does not cause the described symptoms.

D. The peroneal nerve [Correct] travels around the upper aspect of the fibula and can be injured when the bone is fractured. Peroneal nerve supplies the peroneus longus and brevis, both of which permit eversion of the foot.

E. The obturator nerve [Incorrect] does not cause the above symptoms.

14-D

    A. Radical mastectomy is a surgical therapy for breast cancer, in which the entire breast, including the nipple-areolar complex [Incorrect], is resected.

    B. Radical mastectomy is a surgical therapy for breast cancer, in which the entire breast, including the axillary nodes [Incorrect], is resected.

    C. Radical mastectomy is a surgical therapy for breast cancer, in which the entire breast, including the pectoralis minor [Incorrect], is resected.

    D. The pectoralis major [Correct] is removed in a radical mastectomy, but it is not removed in a modified radical mastectomy. Radical mastectomy is rarely performed currently, because more conservative surgery and radiation have proven just as effective while being less disfiguring.

    E. Radical mastectomy is a surgical therapy for breast cancer, in which the entire breast, including the supraclavicular lymph nodes [Incorrect], is resected.

15-E

    A. Never try to insert a Foley catheter [Incorrect] in suspected urethral injury, as it can result in infection, hematoma, or more severe urethral injury.

    B. Scrotal ultrasound [Incorrect] may be done after retrograde urethrogram is performed.

    C. Abdominal/pelvic CT [Incorrect] may be done after retrograde urethrogram is performed.

    D. Abdominal/pelvic MRI [Incorrect] may be done after retrograde urethrogram is performed.

    E. The patient's symptoms are consistent with traumatic rupture of the urethra. The diagnostic modality of choice is the retrograde urethrogram [Correct]. In men, blood at the urethral meatus indicates urethral injury until proven otherwise.

16-C

    A. Portal hypertension secondary to cirrhosis [Incorrect] typically reveals transudative ascites (protein <2.5 g/dl).

    B. Acute pancreatitis [Incorrect] results in elevated amylase and lipase.

    C. This patient has Budd–Chiari syndrome [Correct], which is defined as occlusion of the hepatic veins and/or suprahepatic inferior vena cava, producing postsinusoidal (extrahepatic) portal hypertension that develops secondary to obstruction of hepatic venous drainage. It is characterized by the onset of ascites, abdominal pain, tender hepatomegaly, and protein >2.5 g/dL in ascitic fluid.

D. Portal hypertension secondary to congestive heart failure [Incorrect] typically reveals transudative ascites (protein <2.5 g/dl).

E. Acute splenic rupture [Incorrect] typically occurs due to blunt injury to the abdomen.

17-A

A. Ewing sarcoma [Correct] is the second most common primary bone malignancy affecting children and young adults. Ewing sarcoma can develop in almost any bone or soft tissue, but the most common site is in a flat or long bone, and patients typically present with localized pain and swelling after a history of previous trauma. Typical x-ray findings are poorly marginated destructive lesion, associated soft-tissue mass, "permeative" or "moth-eaten" pattern, and "onion peel" appearance. The "onion peel" appearance is due to periosteal reaction creating layers of reactive bone. Treatment of Ewing sarcoma generally involves surgical resection, chemotherapy, and adjuvant radiotherapy.

B. Osteosarcoma [Incorrect] is the most common primary bone malignancy affecting children and young adults. Characteristic features of osteosarcomas include destruction of the normal trabecular bone pattern, indistinct margins, and no endosteal bone response. The affected bone is characterized by a mixture of radiodense and radiolucent areas, with periosteal new bone formation, lifting of the cortex, and formation of the Codman triangle. The associated soft-tissue mass is variably ossified in a radial or "sunburst" pattern.

C. Hematoma [Incorrect] does not cause bone reactions described above.

D. Rhabdomyosarcoma [Incorrect] does not cause bone reactions described above.

E. Lack of fever and other symptoms rule out osteomyelitis [Incorrect].

18-D

A. An abdominal aneurysm [Incorrect] is not related to trauma and presents as a pulsatile mass.

B. Gastritis [Incorrect] does not account for the mass within his abdomen.

C. Crohn disease [Incorrect] has no relation to trauma and presents in a different manner (fever, diffuse abdominal pain, fistulas, blood per rectum).

D. The presence of epigastric pain, early satiety, and epigastric mass several weeks after trauma to the abdomen is a classic presentation of pancreatic pseudocyst [Correct]. He will likely need surgery (internal drainage) or interventional radiology (external drainage).

E. A persistent colitis [Incorrect] would likely cause fever, continued diarrhea, and pain lower in the abdomen/pelvis.

19-C

A. Urinary tract infection is possible as well, but is less likely in a male, and is more likely to develop on the third postoperative day. Therefore, "urinalysis, urine culture, and antibiotics" [Incorrect] is an incorrect answer.

B. Deep vein thrombosis is also a possibility in this patient, but usually develops about a week after surgery and signs of leg swelling. Therefore, ultrasound of the lower extremities to check for deep vein thrombosis [Incorrect] is not indicated at this time.

C. The most likely cause of fever in the postoperative patient is atelectasis, especially on the first postoperative day. Incentive spirometry can work quite well in alleviating this problem, but requires the participant to be actively using the device. If the atelectasis is not corrected, it can lead to pneumonia, which can be diagnosed with a chest x-ray and treated with the right antibiotics [Correct].

D. Abdominal CT [Incorrect] is an attempt to find an abscess secondary to surgery, which is not consistent with the clinical appearance of the wound and is unlikely to cause a fever the first day after surgery.

E. Reexploratory surgery [Incorrect] is an attempt to find an abscess secondary to surgery, which is not consistent with the clinical appearance of the wound and is unlikely to cause a fever the first day after surgery.

20-A

A. The most likely cause of breathing problems in a patient with penetrating trauma to the chest is a pneumothorax or hemothorax. This corresponds to the physical exam and vital signs. The patient remains clinically stable, so there should be time to get a confirmatory chest x-ray [Correct]. Pneumothorax should be treated with a chest tube. If a patient's vital signs are unstable, a needle thoracostomy should be performed immediately to relieve tension pneumothorax.

B. A patient with a potential pneumothorax should not be sent off of the surgical floor for a CT scan of the chest [Incorrect], in case his clinical state should suddenly deteriorate.

C. Intubation [Incorrect] in this situation may worsen the pneumothorax and cause cardiovascular collapse.

D. IV fluids [Incorrect] are not urgent if a patient has a stable blood pressure and heart rate.

E. A diagnostic peritoneal lavage [Incorrect] is only useful for diagnosing blood or other fluid in the abdominal cavity.

credits

Barash PG, Cullen BF, Stoetling RK. *Clinical Anesthesia.* 5th ed. Philadelphia: Lippincott Williams & Wilkins; 2005. Fig. 19-5 (74-1).

Becker KL, Bilezikian JP, Brenner WJ, et al. *Principles and Practice of Endocrinology and Metabolism.* 3rd ed. Philadelphia: Lippincott Williams & Wilkins; 2001. Figs. 88-5 (8-1), 188-4 (8-2), 40-3 (9-1), 20-2.4 (16-1).

Bhushan V, Le T, Pall V. *Underground Clinical Vignettes: Step 2 Surgery.* 3rd ed. Malden, MA: Blackwell; 2005. Figs. 01A (1-1), 03A (3-1), 12A (13-1), 12B (13-2), 12C (13-3), 12D (13-4), 13A (14-1), 13B (14-2), 13C (14-3), 17A (18-1), 17B (18-2), 17C (18-3), 26A (29-1), 26B (29-2), 29 (31-1), 33A (33-1), 33B (33-2), 33C (33-3), 33D (33-4), 45A (52-1), 45B (52-2), 45C (52-3), 46A (53-1), 46B (53-2), 46C (53-3), 46D (53-4), 49A (54-1), 49B (54-2), 49C (54-3).

Corman ML. *Colon & Rectal Surgery.* 5th ed. Philadelphia: Lippincott Williams & Wilkins; 2004. Figs. 28-44 (7-1), 23-6A (22-1), 22-15 (23-1), 8-29 (30-1), 28-23 (32-1), 28-24 (32-2).

Fleming ID, Cooper JS, Hensen DE, et al., eds. *AJCC Cancer Staging Manual.* Philadelphia: Lippincott–Raven; 1977: 83–90. Table 27-1, Appendix.

Gillenwater JY, Grayhack JT, et al. *Adult and Pediatric Urology.* 4th ed. Philadelphia: Lippincott Williams & Wilkins; 2001. Figs. 3c.42 (44-1), 41.9 (47-1), 53.14 (48-1).

Greenspan A. *Orthopedic Imaging: A Practical Approach.* 4th ed. Philadelphia: Lippincott Williams & Wilkins; 2004. Figs. 5.39 (49-1), 5.42 (49-2), 5.48 (49-3), 5.49 (49-4), 11.78a,b,c (55-1).

Humes HD. *Kelley's Textbook of Internal Medicine.* 2nd ed. Philadelphia: Lippincott Williams & Wilkins; 2001. Figs. 106.4A (11-1), 97.5A (15-1).

Kelsen DP, Daly JM, Kern SE, et al. *Gastrointestinal Oncology: Principles and Practice.* Philadelphia: Lippincott Williams & Wilkins; 2002. Fig. 10.8 (27-2).

Kopans DB. *Breast Imaging.* 3rd ed. Philadelphia: Lippincott Williams & Wilkins; 2006. Figs. 15-1 (36-1), 16-1 (37-1).

MacDonald GM, Seshia MMK, Mullett MD. *Avery's Neonatology: Pathophysiology and Management of the Newborn*. Philadelphia: Lippincott Williams & Wilkins; 2005. Fig. 44.6 (4-1).

Mulholland MW, Lillemoe KD, Doherty GM, et al. *Greenfield's Surgery: Scientific Principles & Practice*. 4th ed. Philadelphia: Lippincott Williams & Wilkins; 2005. Figs. 110.37 (5-1), 110.38 (5-2) 50.3 (6-1), 44-2 (10.1), 60.5 (17-1), 72.26 (20.1), 74.1 (21.2), 73.27 (25-1), 62.13A (26-1), 75.7 (34-1), 113.15a (51-1), 102.3 (56-1), 102.4 (56-2), 92.4 (57.1), 8.1 (72-1), 11.1 (73-1).

Nettina SM. *Lippincott Manual of Nursing Practice*. 8th ed. Philadelphia: Lippincott Williams & Wilkins; 2005. Fig. 7-4 (65-1).

Oldham KT, Colombani PM, et al. *Principles and Practice of Pediatric Surgery*. Philadelphia: Lippincott Williams & Wilkins; 2004. Fig. 71.1B (42-1).

Perkins J, MD. Children's Hospital and Regional Medical Center, Seattle, WA. Courtesy Figs. 70-1, 70-2.

Rowland LP. *Merritt's Neurology*. 11th ed. Philadelphia: Lippincott Williams & Wilkins; 2005. Figs. 63.4 (71-1), 64.5 (75-1).

Schrier RW. *Diseases of the Kidney and Urinary Tract*. 8th ed. Philadelphia: Lippincott Williams & Wilkins; 2006. Fig. 12.7 (35-1).

Sheilds TW, et al. *General Thoracic Surgery*. 6th ed. Philadelphia: Lippincott Williams & Wilkins; 2004. Fig. 128-7 (24-1).

Topol EJ, Califf RM, Isner J, et al. *Textbook of Cardiovascular Medicine*. 2nd ed. Philadelphia: Lippincott Williams & Wilkins; 2002. Figs. 110.3 (64-1), 110.4 (64-2).

Vogelzang NJ, et al. *Comprehensive Textbook of Genitourinary Oncology*. 3rd ed. Philadelphia: Lippincott Williams & Wilkins; 2005. Fig. 22.1 (44-2).

Wolfson AB, Hendey GW, et al. *Harwood-Nuss' Clinical Practice of Emergency Medicine*. 4th ed. Philadelphia: Lippincott Williams & Wilkins; 2005. Fig. 69.2 (6-2).

Yamada T, Alpers DH, et al. *Textbook of Gastroenterology*. 4th ed. Philadelphia: Lippincott Williams & Wilkins; 2003. Figs. 155-5 (6-3), 92-2 (19-1), 153-17 (21-1), 155-5 (27-1), 121-6a,b (31-2), 84-10 (38-1).

case list

PEDIATRIC

1. Atrial Septal Defect
2. Coarctation of the Aorta
3. Tetralogy of Fallot
4. Tracheoesophageal Fistula
5. Pyloric Stenosis

GENERAL SURGERY

6. Small Bowel Obstruction (SBO)
7. Large-Bowel Obstruction (LBO)
8. Pheochromocytoma
9. Thyroid Cancer
10. Boerhaave Syndrome
11. Achalasia
12. Diverticulitis
13. Pancreatic Pseudocyst
14. Acute Pancreatitis
15. Perforated Peptic Ulcer Disease
16. Tension Pneumothorax
17. Portal Hypertension
18. Acute Cholecystitis
19. Anal Fissure
20. Anal Fistula
21. Acute Appendicitis
22. Rectal Cancer
23. Colon Cancer
24. Esophageal Cancer
25. Femoral Hernia
26. Gallstone Ileus
27. Gastric Cancer
28. Upper GI Bleed (UGIB)
29. Lower GI Bleed
30. Hemorrhoids
31. Inguinal Hernia

32. Mesenteric Ischemia
33. Pancreatic Cancer
34. Splenic Rupture
35. Benign Prostatic Hypertrophy
36. Benign Breast Nodule
37. Breast Cancer
38. Crohn Disease
39. Ulcerative Colitis
40. Obstructive Sleep Apnea
41. Zollinger-Ellison Syndrome
42. Meckel Diverticulum
43. Compartment Syndrome

GENITOURINARY

44. Bladder Cancer
45. Prostate Cancer
46. Renal Cell Carcinoma
47. Testicular Cancer
48. Testicular Torsion

ORTHOPEDIC

49. Shoulder Dislocation
50. Dupuytren Contracture
51. Hip Fracture
52. Osteosarcoma
53. Osteomyelitis
54. Radius Fracture
55. Lower Back Pain

VASCULAR

56. Abdominal Aortic Aneurysm
57. Carotid Stenosis
58. Peripheral Vascular Disease

THORACIC
59. Lung Cancer
60. Aortic Dissection

SKIN
61. Melanoma
62. Necrotizing Fasciitis

OPERATIVE CARE/ANESTHESIA
63. Fluid Status
64. Postop Pulmonary Embolism
65. Wound Healing
66. Postop Fever
67. Malignant Hyperthermia

HEAD AND NECK
68. Intracranial Hyptertension
69. Head and Neck Cancer
70. Foreign-Body Aspiration

NEUROLOGY
71. Spinal Cord Compression

TRAUMA
72. Hypovolemic Shock
73. Burns
74. Cervical Spine Injury
75. Head Trauma
76. Chest Trauma

index